HANDBOOK OF VITAMINS AND HORMONES

Roman J. Kutsky, Ph.D.

Associate Professor of Biology
Texas Woman's University
DENTON, TEXAS

VNR **Van Nostrand Reinhold Company**
New York   Cincinnati   Toronto   London   Melbourne

Van Nostrand Reinhold Company Regional Offices:
New York   Cincinnati   Chicago   Millbrae   Dallas
Van Nostrand Reinhold Company International Offices:
London   Toronto   Melbourne
Copyright © 1973 by Litton Educational Publishing, Inc.
Library of Congress Catalog Card Number: 70-190499
ISBN: 0-442-24549-1
Manufactured in the United States of America
Published by Van Nostrand Reinhold Company
450 West 33rd Street, New York, N.Y. 10001
Published simultaneously in Canada by Van Nostrand Reinhold Ltd.
15 14 13 12 11 10 9 8 7 6 5 4 3 2 1

Library of Congress Cataloging in Publication Data

Kutsky, Roman J   1922—
    Handbook of vitamins and hormones.

    Bibliography: p.
    1.   Vitamins.   2.   Vitamin therapy.   3.   Hormones.
4.   Hormone therapy.   I.   Title.
RM259.K88   612'.399   70—190499
ISBN 0—442—24549—1

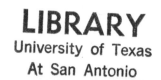

Preface

The properties and modes of action of both the vitamins and the hormones, and their interrelationships to each other as metabolic controlling agents, are easily accessible in this handbook. The book was written to alleviate the continued frustration experienced by many people, including myself, when attempting to obtain unitary, basic information on vitamins and hormones. Although many of the data are separately available, they are so scattered in many compendia, original research papers, and reviews that a small research project on each vitamin and hormone is required before most of the data can be placed in proper context and profitably used. This feeling of dissatisfaction was brought to a head when I recently presented graduate courses in Endocrinology and on Vitamins and Hormones, thus providing the stimulus for this book. Much of the material, and the general format of this volume were generated from lecture notes for the course on Vitamins and Hormones.

It is hoped that this book will be of use to researchers and students in the various fields of life sciences, as well as to physicians, pharmacologists, nurses, and dietitians. Moreover, this book has sufficient content of semitechnical language to make it useful to the educated layman who might need ready information to guide him through the vitamin fads of the day, including rational meal and cooking selections, and to aid in understanding the hormone-related articles in various newspapers and magazines.

I wish to emphasize the fact that conflicting data exist in the various literature sources. The values finally selected, in cases of doubt, were those that could be confirmed by reference to other publications and/or to original literature, where possible. Comments and more recent data are solicited from the readers, especially on individual values and on the format and content of this handbook, as it is my hope to continually improve the usefulness of this volume in future editions.

Many have aided and encouraged me in the preparation of this book. I am grateful to numerous investigators in the fields of nutrition and endocrinology and to my scientific colleagues. In particular I wish to acknowledge the assistance of Dr. Mohamed Aboul-Ela on the sections on plant biosynthesis of vitamins and the aid of Dr. Phyllis Kutsky, my wife, for helpful comments and criticisms and for expediting the final manuscript. My thanks also to Mrs. Bobbie Trietsch for her proficient typing of the manuscript.

I wish to thank the National Academy of Sciences for permission to reproduce the table of RECOMMENDED DAILY DIETARY ALLOWANCES, Seventh Revised Edition, 1968.

Abbreviations

A.A. . . . . amino acid
Absn. . . . . absorption
Acet. . . . . acetone
ACH . . . . acetyl choline
ACTH . . . . . adrenocorticotrop(h)ic
hormone
ADH . . . . antidiuretic hormone
(vasopressin)
Ala. . . . . .alanine
Aldos. . . . . .aldosterone
Alc. . . . .(ethyl) alcohol
Alk. . . . . alkaline
AMP . . . . adenosine monophosphate
cAMP . . . . . . cyclic adenosine mono-
phosphate
Approx. . . . . approximately
Aq. . . . . aqueous
Arg. . . . . arginine
Asn. . . . . .asparagine
Asp. . . . . aspartic acid
ATP . . . . adenosine triphosphate

Benz. . . . . benzene
Bio. . . . . .biotin
BMR . . . . basal metabolic rate

CF . . . . .citrovorum factor
Chl. . . . . chloroform
CHO . . . . .carbohydrate
Chromatog. . . . . chromatograph
CMC, CM cell . . . . . carboxymethyl
cellulose
CNS . . . . . . central nervous system
CoA . . . . coenzyme A
Conc. . . . . .concentrated
Conv. . . . . converted
CoQ . . . . Coenzyme Q
Cort. . . . . .cortisol
CRH . . . . .corticotrop(h)in-releasing
hormone
Cys. . . . . cysteine

DDT . . . dichloro-diphenyl-trichloro-
ethane (insecticide)
DEAE . . . . diethylaminoethyl
(cellulose)
Defic. . . . . .deficiency
Dil. . . . . .dilute
DOPA . . . . dihydroxyphenylalanine
DPN . .diphosphopyridine nucleotide
DNA . . . . deoxyribonucleic acid

Enz. . . . . enzyme

Ep., Epi. . . . . .epinephrine
Equiv. . . . . .equivalent
Esp. . . . . especially
Est. . . . . estradiol
Eth. . . . . ether
Ext. . . . . extract

F.A. . . . . folic acid
FAD . . . .flavin adenine dinucleotide
FMN . . . . .flavin mononucleotide
FRH . . . . . . FSH-releasing hormone
FSH . . . .follicle-stimulating hormone
Fluoresc. . . . . fluorescent

GH . . . . growth hormone (STH)
G.I. . . . . gastro-intestinal
Gln. . . . . .glutamine
Glu. . . . . .glutamic acid
Gluc(ag). . . . . .glucagon
Gly. . . . . .glycine
GPU . . . . .guinea pig unit
GRH . . . . growth (somatotrop(h)in)
releasing hormone

HCG . . . . .human chorionic gonado-
trophin
HGH . . . . . human growth hormone
His. . . . . .histidine
HMG . human menopause gonadotro-
phin (mixture of FSH and LH)
HMP . . . . . . hexose monophosphate
Hyp. R.F., HRH . hypothalamic-releas-
ing factor (hormone)

Ile. . . . . isoleucine
In. . . . . insulin
Insol. . . . . .insoluble
IRC . . . . ion exchange resin
Irrad. . . . . irradiated
I.U. . . . . international unit
I.V. . . . . intravenous

Leu. . . . . .leucine
LH . . . . luteinizing hormone
LLD . . . . L. lactis Dorner
LRH . . . . . . .LH-releasing hormone
Lys. . . . . .lysine

Max. . . . . .maximum
me. . . . . .methyl
Met. . . . . methionine
Metab. . . . . .metabolism
MIH . . . . . MSH-inhibiting hormone
Monocl. . . . . monoclinic
MP . . . . .melting point
MRH . . . . . .MSH-releasing hormone
MSH melanocyte-stimulating hormone
MW . . . . molecular weight

NAD(P) . . . nicotinamide adenine di-
nucleotide (phosphate)
NADPH . . . . .reduced NADP
Nia. . . . . .niacin
NIH . . . National Institutes of Health
Nor., Norepi. . . . . . . norepinephrine
NRC . . . . National Research Council

OAA . . . . .oxaloacetic acid
Oxy. . . . . .oxytocin

P.A., Pant. . . . . . . pantothenic acid
PBI . . . . protein-bound iodine
Pet. . . . . .petroleum
PGA . . . .pteroyl glutamic acid, folic
acid
Phe . . . . .phenylalanine
pI . . . . .isoelectric point
PIH . . . prolactin-inhibiting hormone
PMSG . . . . . . .pregnant mare serum
gonadotrophin
Ppt. . . . . precipitate
PRH . . . prolactin-releasing hormone
Pro. . . . . .proline
Prog. . . . . progesterone

Prol. . . . . .prolactin
PTH . . . . parathormone

RBC . . . . red blood cell
Relax. . . . . relaxin
RNA . . . . ribonucleic acid
_mRNA . . . messenger ribonucleic acid

Ser. . . . . .serine
Serot. . . . . serotonin
Sl. . . . . .slightly
Sol. . . . . .soluble
Soln. . . . . solution
Std. . . . . standard
STH . . . . somatotrop(h)in (GH)

T3 . . . . triiodothyronine
T4 . . .tetraiodothyronine (thyroxine)

TCA . . . . tricarboxylic acid (cycle),
        Krebs (cycle)
TCT . . . . thyrocalcitonin
Test., Testos. . . . . testosterone
Thr. . . . . threonine
TPN . . triphosphopyridine nucleotide
        (NADP)
TRH . . . . . . TSH-releasing hormone
Try. . . . . tryptophan
TSH . . . thyroid-stimulating hormone
Tyr. . . . . tyrosine

UDP . . . . uridine diphosphate
USP . . . .*United States Pharmacopeia*
UV . . . . .ultraviolet

Val. . . . . .valine
Vaso. . . . . vasopressin
Vit. . . . . .vitamin

Contents

1
Introduction

With the new discoveries in molecular biology, biochemistry, physiology, and endocrinology, the emphasis in research in life sciences is turning from descriptive biochemistry and electron microscopy to the functional, dynamic aspects of the vital, metabolic processes. In particular, great interest has been generated in the actual controlling agents which accurately blend all the cellular enzyme systems and organelles to produce a living cell, and, from that, a living multicellular organism. It is precisely in this area of control mechanisms that the vitamins and hormones play such a key role, because they are controlling agents.

This book is written primarily from the standpoint of the vitamin and hormone requirements and contents of individuals of the *human* species. It should be understood that requirements and contents differ from species to species, in general becoming simpler as one goes down the evolutionary scale. For the purposes of this book, a *vitamin* is defined as a biologically active, organic compound, a controlling agent essential for an organism's (human's) normal health and growth (its absence causing a deficiency disease or disorder), not synthesized within the organism, available in the diet in small amounts, and carried in the circulatory system in small concentrations to act on target organs or tissues. A *hormone* is defined as a biologically active, organic compound, a controlling agent essential for normal health and growth (its absence causing a deficiency disease or disorder), synthesized within the organism (human being) in ductless glands which release the agent in very small concentrations into the circulatory system to act on the target organs or tissues.

The chief differences between a vitamin and a hormone seem to be the site of biosynthesis, the types of organic compounds present in vitamins as opposed to the hormones, and some of the modes of action. These differences between

1

vitamins and hormones in essential properties are small compared to their similarities and explain why both vitamins and hormones are combined into one book.

In the light of new evidence, it is becoming difficult to differentiate certain vitamins from some hormones. For example, both vitamin D and niacin are synthesized (but in an inadequate amount) in the human, thus conferring on them a hormonal quality. Similarly, the human requirement for the hormone thyroxine can be partially satisfied by a dietary intake of iodine, and some of the steroid hormones are active in a dietary form thus giving them a vitamin quality. Moreover, the fat-soluble vitamins (A, D, E, K) show many similarities in biosynthesis, structure, properties and function to the fat-soluble hormones (steroids). Finally, the same molecule can function as a hormone or as a vitamin depending on the species involved. For example, vitamin C functions as a vitamin in primates because they cannot synthesize it, but it functions as a hormone in rats because they can synthesize it.

We can see that the concept of vitamins and hormones, as defined here, could be extended to all organisms with circulatory systems and would therefore include all vertebrates, many invertebrates, and the higher plants, excepting mainly the lower plants and animals and unicellular organisms. If the definition of circulatory system were to include intracellular circulation, then all living organisms would be included. The concept of vitamin is therefore very much dependent on the species concerned as, if we accept the expanded definition of circulatory system, then the "vitamins" synthesized by unicellular organisms would actually be hormones. Vitamins seem to have arisen very early in the evolution of life as judged by their presence and requirement in some of the most primitive forms of life known today. Hormones, according to our original definition, however, denote a much later period of emergence, becoming prominent mainly with the evolution of the various animals. They, therefore, reflect a shorter evolutionary history. In view of their primitive nature, vitamins would be expected to have, in general, a simpler structure than hormones, and this is indeed the case, with a few exceptions.

As we compare modes of action of vitamins and hormones, we should compare their chemical structures. The vitamins consist of a fat-soluble series and a water-soluble series. The fat-soluble vitamins (A, D, E, K) consist of derivatives of partially cyclized isoprenoid polymers, somewhat similar to the intermediates in cholesterol (steroid) synthesis. These vitamins seem to act by virtue of their lipid solubility in various cell membranes to affect permeability or transport, and by virtue of their chemical groups as redox agents (A, E, K), as coenzymes or enzyme activators (D, K, A), or as enzyme inhibitors (E). The water-soluble vitamins (B_1, B_2, B_6, B_{12}, niacin, pantothenic acid, folic acid, biotin, C) consist, in general, of derivatives or substituted derivatives of sugars (C), pyridine (niacin, B_6), purines and pyrimidines (folic acid, B_2, B_1), amino acid-organic acid complexes (folic acid, biotin, pantothenic acid) and a porphyrin-nucleotide complex (B_{12}). These structurally diverse water-soluble vitamins act as enzyme activators and coenzymes (B_1, B_2, B_6, B_{12}, pantothenic acid, folic acid, biotin, niacin), as redox agents on enzyme reactions (C, B_2, B_{12}, folic acid, niacin) as nuclear agents (folic acid, B_{12}, C, biotin) and probably mitochondrial agents (B_2, C, niacin).

The hormones also include a fat-soluble, steroid series (estradiol, progesterone, aldosterone, testosterone, cortisol) which seems to act (1) by virtue of lipid solubility to stabilize and change permeability of the cell membranes, (2) to regulate enzyme activity and membrane polarization, (3) to regulate redox potential, and (4) to affect RNA transcription in the nucleus (aldosterone, estradiol, testosterone). The water-soluble hormones consist of a protein series (STH, TSH, FSH, LH, Prol.) which seems to act on the cell membrane to stimulate cyclic AMP production with consequent ATP production, and enzyme activation, and to activate certain genes in the nucleus. The peptide series of water-soluble hormones (insulin, glucagon, ACTH, MSH, oxytocin, ADH, PTH, T4, TCT, and relaxin) acts similarly to the proteins and also has an effect on the mitochondria by T4 and PTH. The amine, water-soluble hormone series (epinephrine, norepinephrine) seems to act chiefly by the cyclic AMP mechanism on the membrane, with consequent enzyme activation. The very extensive role of $_c$AMP as an intracellular mediator of hormonal activity is most noteworthy.

It can be seen that the fat-soluble vitamins and hormones act similarly on membranes, on redox potentials, and as enzyme activators, the only difference being in a demonstrated action on the nucleus by the steroids. Comparison of the water-soluble series of hormones with that of the vitamins again shows a basic similarity in action, the vitamins acting as direct enzyme activators and coenzymes, and the hormones acting as indirect activators via cyclic AMP. Both act on the nucleus but differ in that only some of the water-soluble vitamins have redox properties. Again here, the differences between the two water-soluble series of vitamins and hormones lie chiefly in their differing structures and in some of their properties, such as redox regulation and presence of cyclic AMP intermediates.

The subject of vitamin requirements requires comment. There is now sufficient evidence to indicate that the concept of biochemical individuality has much merit. Thus the recommended allowances as stated in this book (NRC Data) should be considered only as average figures, and variations (increase or decrease) of twentyfold or more in individual human requirements may be found, depending on the genetic and physiological state of the individual. Germane to this are the topics of subclinical vitamin deficiencies and megavitamin therapy, i.e., large overdosages of one or more vitamins such as are now being used as treatment of colds and schizophrenia.

The existence of subclinical vitamin deficiencies is extremely difficult to prove without adequate statistical data, but, undoubtedly, if we accept the principle of biochemical individuality, they do exist. In like manner, the use of megavitamins may be helpful to those individuals whose systems for some reason destroy these vitamins rapidly or require these vitamins in large quantity due to their biochemical individuality. However, in view of the fact that accurate data are lacking, megavitamins should be treated and used as drugs with competent medical advice, being wary of possible unexpected individual toxicity.

A perusal of the miscellaneous section for each hormone or vitamin will indicate to the reader the enormous amount of interplay occurring among vitamins and hormones themselves and also with each other. This includes both antagonisms and synergisms occurring simultaneously among various vitamins and hormones. Undoubtedly there exists an optimal set of levels for each vitamin and hormone which, presumably, is that which has been found in "normal" human values. But maximum optimization of levels at "normal" human values has not been proven experimentally; perhaps the human system could run more efficiently at a different set of values. More research is needed to determine this. In any case, optimum amounts and ratios of all vitamins and hormones are important to get full benefits of these agents.

Lack of space and time has precluded extensive mention of the trace elements and mineral cofactors required for functioning of most coenzyme systems as well as some hormones, e.g., magnesium, iron, copper, iodine, selenium, cobalt, etc. These trace elements should be present in correct amounts and ratios in any balanced diet containing adequate vitamins.

In relation to requirements, the subject of undiscovered or unaccepted vitamins and hormones should be mentioned. This book has included only those vitamins and hormones with widespread acceptance. In addition to the 13 vitamins listed here, there are at least another 13 compounds with various acceptabilities as vitamins, plus possibly other vitamins still undiscovered. In relationship to individual requirements, this means that taken together with the facts of mutual interdependence of vitamins as mentioned above, it would still be advisable to rely for one's vitamin requirement chiefly on rich natural sources in the diet, since these would most likely contain the undiscovered vitamins. However, in view of the possible extreme losses of vitamin potency even in our richest dietary sources caused by our present methods of processing, storing, and cooking of food, it would be advisable to consider vitamin supplementation of certain vitamins, especially if one's diet has not been carefully planned.

As far as the hormones are concerned, at least another 23 compounds, in addition to the 23 listed here, are known with various degrees of acceptance as true hormones. No doubt many more remain to be discovered. This book has not listed the insect or plant hormones, because the human requirements and levels are being stressed.

2
Presentation
of Data

This book will serve as a ready reference to four major groups of readers, inasmuch as the data for each vitamin and hormone are presented in several separate sections, as follows: "General Information" and "Miscellaneous Information" for the general reader and all other groups; "Medical and Biological Role" mainly for the biologists, physicians, nurses, and pharmacologists; "Chemical Properties" and "Metabolic Properties" for the biochemists and physiologists; and "Nutritional Role" for dietitians and nutritionists. However, it is hoped that parts of all sections will be useful to all the groups. Insofar as possible, the format is similar for both hormones and vitamins for ease of reference. A list of abbreviations is given at the beginning of the book.

The specific vitamins and hormones chosen for coverage in this book are those that have the widest acceptance by the various workers in both fields. Only the most active of the steroid hormones in each category of mineralocorticoids, glucocorticoids, and sex hormones in the human is being covered (out of the 40 plus already discovered).

Chapters on Vitamins and Hormones
General Information Section
"Active analogs and related compounds" includes vitamers, isotels, etc.
"Antagonists" and "Synergists" may be the same chemical species but in different concentrations. Interaction at the target site is used as a criterion of antagonism or synergism.
"Sources for Species" (Essentiality) indicates degree of requirement for various species including man. Endogenous = made within organism. Exogenous sources include intestinal bacteria.

Chemical Properties Section

"Reactions" refers to those carried out with standard laboratory conditions and reagents and not under extreme conditions, unless otherwise noted. i.e., heat $\leqslant 100°C$, weak acids or alkalies, reactivity with water, atmospheric or mild oxidation agents, mild reducing agents, bright daylight.

Isolation method gives a typical procedure now in use.

Medical and Biological (Nutritional) Section

This provides, in general, clinical information. Contents of vitamins are per 100 g. edible portion

Antigenicity is defined as the ability to act as an antigen creating an immune response when administered to an organism. Specificity is here defined as the degree of restriction of biological activity to a certain species.

Metabolic Role Section

"Enzyme Reactions" lists enzyme systems affected by the vitamin or hormone, organ location, and effects on enzymes, where known.

"Mode of Action" subdivides functions on both a cellular basis (anabolic, catabolic, etc.) and an organismal basis. Anabolic denotes synthetic processes; catabolic denotes degredative reactions and includes most energy yielding reactions.

Miscellaneous Information Section

"Relationships to other Vitamins, Hormones" attempts to indicate the mutual involvement of both vitamins and hormones in most actions of both groups either together or within the group.

"Unusual Features" includes various chemical, biological, and pharmacological features that could not be listed elsewhere.

"Possible Relationships" attempts to draw a parallel between the action of vitamin or a hormone and its deficiency symptoms.

The tables following Chapter 38 list in tabular fashion some of the data already presented and some new data in an attempt to indicate fundamental similarities and dissimilarities in structure and function of both vitamins and hormones.

References are presented in numbered form at the end of the book, and are subdivided into three categories: General; Specific: Vitamins; and Specific: Hormones. An effort has been made to cite only the latest available handbooks, compendia, journal references, and texts.

3
Vitamin A

GENERAL INFORMATION

1. **Synonyms:** Retinol, axerophthol, biosterol, vitamin A_1, anti-xerophthalmic vitamin, anti-infective vitamin

2. **History**
   - 1912—Hopkins reported factor in milk needed for growth of rats
   - 1913—Osborne and Mendel demonstrated milk factor is fat soluble; present in other fats also
   - 1913-15—McCollum and Davis identified milk factor (fat-soluble A) in butter, egg yolk
   - 1917—McCollum and Simmonds found xerophthalmia in rats due to lack of fat-soluble A
   - 1920—Drummond renamed fat-soluble A, vit. A
   - 1930—Moore determined carotene a precursor for vit. A
   - 1930-37—Karrer *et al.* isolated and synthesized vit. A
   - 1935—Wald reported visual purple in retina a complex of protein and vit. A

3. **Physiological Forms**
   Retinol (vit. A_1) and esters
   3-Dehydroretinol (vit. A_2) and esters
   Retinal (retinene, vit. A aldehyde), 3-dehydroretinal (retinine-2)
   Retinoic acid
   Neovitamin A
   Neo-b-vit. A_1

4. **Active Analogs and Related Compounds:** α, β, γ-carotene, neo-β-carotene B, cryptoxanthine, myxoxanthine, torularhodin, aphanicin, echinenone

5. **Inactive Analogs and Related Compounds:**   Kitol, xanthophyll, lycopene

6. **Antagonists:**   Sodium benzoate, bromobenzene, citral, oxidized derivatives of vit. A, thyroxine (large concentrations), estrogens, vitamin E (membrane permeability)

7. **Synergists:**   Vitamins B_2, B_{12}, C, E, thyroxine, testosterone, MSH, STH

8. **Physiological Functions:**   Growth, production of visual purple, maintenance of skin and epithelial cells, resistance to infection, gluconeogenesis, mucopolysaccharide synthesis, bone development, maintenance of myelin and membranes, maintenance of color and peripheral vision, maintenance of adrenal cortex and steroid hormone synthesis

9. **Deficiency Diseases, Disorders:**   Xerophthalmia, nyctalopia, hemeralopia, keratomalacia, hyperkeratosis

10. **Sources for Species Requiring It**
    Required by many animal species
    Exogenous sources—All vertebrates and some invertebrates convert plant dietary carotenoids in gut to vit. A_1, which is absorbed
    Endogenous sources—None reported

CHEMISTRY

1. **Structure**

Vitamin A_1, $C_{20}H_{30}O$

β-ionone

2. **Reactions**

    Heat—Labile (isomerizes)
    Acid—Labile (isomerizes)
    Alkali—Stable
    Water—Insol.

    Oxidation—Labile (isomerizes)
    Reduction—Stable
    Light—Labile (isomerizes) (UV
        inactivates)

3. **Properties**

    Appearance—Yellow oil
    MW—286.4
    MP—62-64°C
    Crystal Form—Prisms
    Salts, Esters—Acetate palmitate
    Important Groups for activity
      β-ionone ring
      trans-methyl
      Alcoholic hydroxyl

    Solubility
      H_2O—Insol.
      Acet., Alc.—Sol.
      Chl., Eth.—Sol.
    Absn. Max.—325-328 mμ
    Chemical Nature—Unsaturated alc.
    $\alpha_D = 0$ (inactive)

4. **Commercial Production**

    Chemical—Extraction of fish liver
    Synthetic—From citral or β-ionone

5. **Isolation**

    Sources—Fish liver oils
    Method—Saponification in alcoholic KOH. Extract with ether, crystallize

6. **Determination**

    Bioassay—Growth rate of rats
    Physicochemical—Spectrophotometric determination of blue color on
        reacting with antimony trichloride or trifluoracetic acid

DISTRIBUTION AND SOURCES

1. **Occurrence**

    Plants
        Fruit—Provitamin carotenoids—apricots, yellow melons, peaches,
            prunes
        Vegetables—Provitamin carotenoids—beet greens, broccoli greens,
            carrots, endive, kale, lettuce, mint, mustard, parsley, pumpkins,
            spinach, sweet potatoes, turnip greens, cress
        Nuts—Provitamin carotenoids—in small quantity in most nuts

Animals:
  Vitamin A in all vertebrates, and carotenoids in certain invertebrates
    (crustacea) (A_2 especially in fresh-water fish)
  Location: Liver, heart, lungs, fat, adrenals, retina, kidney, milk, blood
    plasma, egg
  Provitamin carotenoids found in many animals depending on diet
  Hen's egg carotenoid mainly xanthophyll (inactive analog)
  Microorganisms: Provitamin carotenoids in algae, fungi, bacteria. No
    intestinal synthesis of vit. A

2. **Dietary Sources:**   (Vit. A and Procarotenoids)
  High: 10,000–76,000 I.U./100 g
    Liver (beef, pig, sheep, calf, chicken)
    Liver oil (cod, halibut, salmon, shark, sperm whale)
    Carrots, mint, kohlrabi, parsley, spinach, turnip greens, dandelion
      greens, palm oil
  Medium: 1000-10,000 I.U./100 g
    Butter, cheese (except cottage), egg yolk, margarine, dried milk, cream
    White fish, eel
    Kidneys (beef, pig, sheep), liver (pork)
    Mangoes, apricots, yellow melons, peaches, cherries (sour), nectarines
    Beet greens, broccoli, endive, kale, mustard, pumpkin, sweet
      potatoes, watercress, tomatoes, leek greens, chicory, chives,
      collards, fennel, butterhead and romaine lettuce, squash (acorn,
      butternut, hubbard), chard
  Low: 100-1000 I.U./100 g
    Milk
    Herring, salmon, oyster, carp, clams, sardines
    Grapes, bananas, berries (black-, goose-, rasp-, boysen-, logan-, blue-),
      sweet cherries, olives, oranges, avocados, prunes, kumquats, pine-
      apples, plums, rhubarb, tangerines, red currants
    Summer and zucchini squash, asparagus, beans (except kidney),
      brussel sprouts, cabbages, leeks, peas, artichokes, corn, cucumbers,
      lentils (dry), peppers, lettuce, celery, cowpeas, rutabagas, okra
    Hazelnuts, peanuts, black walnuts, cashew, pecans, pistachios

MEDICAL AND NUTRITIONAL ROLE

1. **Units:**   1 I.U. = 0.344 μg vit. A acetate = 0.3 μg retinol

2. **Normal Blood Levels:**   100-300 I.U./100 ml serum

3. **Recommended Allowances**
   Children—2000-3500 I.U./day
   Adults—5000 I.U./day
   Special—Pregnancy—6000 I.U./day, Lactation—8000 I.U./day

4. **Administration**
   Injection—Parenteral
   Topical—No data
   Oral—Preferred route

5. **Factors Affecting Availability**
   Decrease
   Liver damage
   Impaired intestinal conversion of carotenes
   Impaired absorption (low bile)
   Food preparation (cooking and frying—heat oxidation)
   Presence of antagonists
   Illness—increased destruction and excretion
   Increase
   Storage in body (liver)
   Intestinal conversion of carotenes—T4, insulin increase
   Absorption aids—bile, fat
   Dietary protein—mobilizes Vit. A from storage in liver

6. **Deficiency Symptoms**
   General
   Retarded growth
   Night blindness (nyctalopia)—degeneration of retina
   Hyperkeratinization of epithelial tissues—
   Degenerative changes in eye epithelium (xerophthalmia, hemeralopia)
   Atrophy of odontoblasts
   Lab animals
   Poor bone and tooth development
   Resorption of fetus, atrophy of germinal epithelium
   Urolithiasis—urinary calculi

7. **Effects of Overdose**
   100,000 units/day (man)—generally toxic
   Irritability, nerve lesions
   Fatigue, insomnia, painful bones and joints
   Exophthalmia
   Mucous cell formation in keratinized membranes

Abnormal bone growth
Loss of hair, jaundice, itchy skin, anorexia
Decreased clotting time
Elevated serum alkaline phosphatase

METABOLIC ROLE

1. **Biosynthesis**
   Precursors
   Animals—Carotenoid conversion
   (except rat, pig, sheep, carnivores, some invertebrates and human
   infants)—cannot convert
   α, β, γ-carotenes, cryptoxanthin, myxoxanthin, torularhodin
   Plants—Cholesterol pathways—acetate, etc., aphanicin, echinenone
   Intermediates
   Plants—Mevalonic acid, squalene

2. **Production:** Species and sites
   Plants (carotenoids)
   Higher plants—Green leaves, yellow vegetables and fruits
   Some algae, fungi, bacteria—carotenoids
   Animals
   Most vertebrates (except rat, pig, sheep)
   Conversion of carotenoids to vit. A in intestinal wall
   Some invertebrates also convert

3. **Storage Sites:** Liver, kidney (rat, cat)

4. **Blood Carriers**
   α_1 and α_2-globulins, β-lipoproteins (carotenoids)
   Retinol esters via lymphatics (esp. palmitate)
   chylomicrons in lymphatics (retinol esters)

5. **Half-life:** Weeks or months

6. **Target Tissues:** Retina, skin, bone, liver, adrenals, germinal epithelium

7. Reactions

Coenzyme forms—Neo-b-vit. A_1, retinoic acid

Organ	Enzyme System	Effect
Adrenal cortex	Hydroxylating—deoxycorticosterone → corticosterone	Activated
Liver	Sulfurylases—ATP + SO_4 = phospho-adenosinephosphosulfate	Activated
Intestine	Esterases—Vitamin A ester → vit. A + fatty acid	Activated
Intestine	Synthetases—Vit. A + Fatty acid → vit. A ester	Activated
Liver	Dehydrogenases—neo-b-vit. A_1 → retinene, retinal → retinoic acid	Activated
Retina	Isomerases—*trans*-retinene → *cis*-retinene (inactive)	Activated
Liver	Hydrolases—Acid phosphatase, β-glucuro-nidase, cathepsin, etc., in lysosomes on hyper- or hypo-vitaminosis A	Released

8. Mode of Action

Cellular

Anabolic—Synthesis of mucopolysaccharides via "active" sulfate. Synthesis of corticosterone

Catabolic—No data

Other—Precursor of retinene in retina—forms visual pigments. Maintains stability of lysosomes + cell membranes

Organismal

Maintenance of visual sense organs

Maintains reproductive systems

Maintains glucocorticoid production in adrenals

Maintains mucous membranes

Regulates cartilage for bone development

9. Catabolism

Intermediates—Retinoic acid

Excretion products

Urine—Vitamin A (only in disease)

fatty acid, small soluble molecules

Breath—CO_2

MISCELLANEOUS

1. **Relationship to Other Vitamins**

    Vitamin C—Plasma vit. C levels drop on depletion of vit. A, occurrence and action of vits. A and C coincide often

    Vitamin D—Occurs naturally with vit. A in animal liver oils. Toxic overdose effects reduced by vit. A

    Niacin—Involved with DPN + vit. A in activity of retinene reductase.

    Vitamin E—Decreases serum cholesterol in rabbit when given with vit. A
    Protects vit. A from oxidation
    Similarity of structure to vitamin A
    Antagonistic to vit. A in maintaining membrane permeability

    Pantothenic acid—Promotes synthesis of vit. A in plants

2. **Relationship to Hormones**

    Thyroxine—Stimulates intestinal conversion of carotene to vit. A
    Increases vit. A storage in liver
    Antagonizes decreased basal metabolism caused by vit. A
    Increases use of vit. A

    Insulin—Stimulates intestinal conversion of carotene to vit. A

    STH—A synergist in growth

    Cortisol, Aldosterone, Testosterone, Progesterone—Decreased on vit. A depletion (chemical adrenalectomy). Production of deoxycortico-sterone and other steroids stimulated by vit. A

    Estradiol—Antagonistic to vit. A peripherally

    MSH—Decreases dark adaptation time—synergistic to vit. A

3. **Unusual Features**

    Decreases serum cholesterol in large quantity administration (chicks)
    Dietary protein required to mobilize liver reserves of vit. A
    Decreased in tumors
    Coenzyme Q_{10} accumulates in A-deficient rat liver
    Ubichromenol-50 accumulation in A-deficient rat liver
    Retinoic acid functions as vit. A except for visual and reproductive functions
    Anti-infection properties and anti-allergic properties
    Decreases basal metabolism
    Detoxification of poisons in the liver aided by vit. A
    Involved in triose $\rightarrow$ glucose conversions

4. **Possible Relationships of Deficiency Symptoms to Metabolic Action**
Growth Retardation—Effects on steroid synthesis, bone growth, and membrane structure, and development of epithelial tissues
Keratinization—Effects on membranes and mucopolysaccharide biosynthesis
Bone development—Formation of chondroitin sulfate in cartilage
Reproductive failure—Effects on membranes and steroid hormones
Visual defects—Absence of retinene precursors

4
Vitamin D

GENERAL INFORMATION

1. **Synonyms:** Antirachitic vitamin, vitamin D_3, rachitamin, rachitasterol, cholecalciferol, activated 7-dehydrocholesterol

2. **History**
   - 1918—Mellanby produced experimental rickets in dogs
   - 1919—Huldschinsky ameliorated rachitic symptoms in children with ultraviolet irradiation
   - 1922—Hess showed liver oils contain same antirachitic factor as sunlight
   - 1922—McCollum increased calcium deposition in rachitic rats with cod liver oil factor
   - 1924—Steenbock and Hess demonstrated irradiated foods have antirachitic properties
   - 1925—McCollum named antirachitic factor vit. D.
   - 1931—Angus isolated crystalline vit. D (calciferol)
   - 1936—Windaus isolated vit. D_3 (activated 7-dehydrocholesterol)

3. **Physiological Forms:** Vitamin D_2 (calciferol, ergocalciferol), vit. D_3 (cholecalciferol), phosphate esters of D_2, D_3, 25-hydroxycholecalciferol, 1,25-dihydroxycholecalciferol, 5,25-dihydroxycholecalciferol

4. **Active Analogs and Related Compounds:** Irrad. [22-dihydroergosterol (vit. D_4) 2-dehydrostigmasterol (vit. D_6), 7-dehydrositosterol (vit. D_5)]. Dihydrotachysterol

5. **Inactive Analogs and Related Compounds:**   Lumisterol, tachysterol, ergosterol, 7-dehydrocholesterol

6. **Antagonists:**   Toxisterol, phytin, phlorizin, cortisone, cortisol, thyrocalcitonin, PTH

7. **Synergists:**   Niacin, PTH, STH

8. **Physiological Functions:**   Normal growth (via bone growth), Ca and P absorption from intestine, antirachitic, increases tubular P reabsorption, increases citrate blood levels, maintains and activates alkaline phosphatase in bone, and maintains serum calcium and phosphorus levels

9. **Deficiency Diseases, Disorders:**   Rickets, osteomalacia, hypoparathyroidism

10. **Sources for Species Requiring It:**   Required by vertebrates
    Exogenous sources—Infant vertebrates and deficient adult vertebrates
    Endogenous sources—Vertebrates (synthesized in skin under UV irrad.)

CHEMISTRY

1. **Structure**

Vitamin D_3, $C_{27}H_{44}O$

2. **Reactions**

Heat—Stable	Oxidation—Unstable
Acid—Stable	Reduction—Stable
Alkali—Stable	Light—Unstable
Water—Insol.	

3. Properties
   Appearance—White powder
   MW—384.65
   MP—84-85°C
   Form—Fine needles
   Salts, Esters
      Palmitate, 3,5-dinitrobenzoate
   Important Groups for Activity
      $C_{10}-C_{18}$ Methylene
      Alcoholic—OH

   Solubility
      H_2O—Insol.
      Acet., Alc.—Sol.
      Benz., Chl., Eth.—Sol.

   Absn. Max.—265 mμ
   Chemical Nature—Sterol, alc.
   $\alpha_D^{20} = +102.5°$ (alc.)

4. Commercial Production
   Irradiation of ergosterol, 7-dehydrocholesterol
   Extraction of fish liver oils

5. Isolation
   Sources—Liver oil, irradiated yeast
   Method—Saponify oil, remove vit. A and sterols by partitioning solvents,
      and adsorption chromatography, remove inactive sterols with
      digitonin, crystallize as 3,5-dinitrobenzoate ester, saponify, recrys-
      tallize

6. Determination
   Bioassay—Antirachitic test on rats
   Physicochemical—Reaction with antimony trichloride

DISTRIBUTION AND SOURCES

1. Occurrence
   Plants
      Fruit—None
      Vegetables—Grain and vegetable oils (provitamins)
      Nuts—None
   Animals: Tuna, halibut, cod liver oils
      Egg yolk, milk (irrad.), bones, intestine, blood, brain, skin, spleen, fish
         liver
      Shrimp, mollusks
   Microorganisms: Yeast, algae, bacteria (provitamins)

2. Dietary Sources
   High: $1000\text{-}25 \times 10^6$ I.U./100 g
      Liver oils (bonito, tuna, lingcod, sea bass, swordfish, halibut, herring, cod, sablefish, soupfin shark)
   Medium: 100-1000 I.U./100 g
      Egg yolk, margarine, lard, herring, salmon, mackerel, pilchards, sardines, shrimp, tuna, kippers
   Low: 10-100 I.U./100 g
      Grain and vegetable oils
      Cod roe, halibut
      Butter, cream, eggs, cheeses, milk (vit. D or irrad.)
      Liver (calf, pork, lamb, beef)
      Veal, horse meat, beef

MEDICAL AND NUTRITIONAL ROLE

1. **Units:**   1 U.S.P. = 1 I.U. = 0.025 μg vit. D_3

2. **Normal Blood Levels:**   2.75 μg/100 ml (serum); 66-165 I.U./100 ml (serum)

3. **Recommended Allowances**
   Children—400 I.U./day
   Adults—None in equatorial zones; 400 I.U./day in temperate zones (available in normal diet)
   Special—Pregnancy, 400 I.U./day; lactation, 400 I.U./day; senility, night workers, miners, northern people

4. **Administration**
   Injection—Subcutaneous, intraperitoneal, intramuscular (D_3 esters)
   Topical—Absorbed through skin
   Oral—Preferred route

5. **Factors Affecting Availability**
   Decrease
      Liver damage
      Presence of antagonists
      Presence of phytin in gut
      Low bile salts in gut

High pH in gut
Destruction by intestinal flora
Excretion in feces
Increase
Storage in liver, skin
Absorption aids—bile salts
Long acting feature (slow destruction)
Decrease in pH of lower intestine
Irradiation by UV

6. **Deficiency Symptoms**

In young or experimental animals, including man
Retarded growth—Rickets
Malformation of long bones—Rickets
Skeletal malformation
Demineralization of bone
Decreased blood calcium and phosphorus
Increased serum alkaline phosphatase

7. **Effects of Overdose (Man)**—Generally toxic
4000 (or more) I.U./day
Anorexia, nausea, thirst, diarrhea
Polyuria, muscular weakness, joint pains
Increased serum calcium—calcification of soft tissues (arteries, muscle)
Resorption of bone
Arterial lesions and kidney injury (rats)

METABOLIC ROLE

1. **Biosynthesis**
Precursors—Cholesterol (skin—UV) animals; ergosterol (algae, yeast-UV) plants
Intermediates—Pre-ergocalciferol, tachysterol, 7-dehydrocholesterol

2. **Production:**   Species and Site
Plants—Leaves, seeds, shoots (provitamins)
Fungi—Various
Bacteria—Various, but no intestinal synthesis
Animals—Skin

3. **Storage Sites:**   Animals—Liver, skin

4. **Blood Carriers:** Lipoproteins $(\alpha + \beta)$

5. **Half-life:** Long acting (days, weeks)

6. **Target Tissues:** Kidney, bone, intestine, liver

7. **Reactions**
   Reactive form—25-Hydroxycholecalciferol and metabolites
   Coenzyme forms—Phosphorylated vit. D

Organ	Enzyme System	Effect
Intestine	Phytase	Activated
Serum	Alk. phosphatase—Organic phosphate (serum) → inorganic phosphate	Activated
Liver	Phosphorylase—Glycogen → glucose-1-phosphate	Activated

8. **Mode of Action**
   Cellular
   Anabolic—Increases protein synthesis in intestinal cells
   Catabolic
   Depresses protein synthesis except in intestinal cells
   Other
   Decreases citrate oxidation
   Increases release of calcium by mitochondria
   Activates active transport of calcium by intestinal cells
   Repair of mitochondrial membrane
   Regulates phosphorus metabolism
   Organismal
   Promotes normal bone calcification
   Increases formation of osteoclasts and capillaries in cartilage—
   Increases cartilage degeneration in normal bone calcification
   Regulates phosphorus and calcium metabolism—increases calcium
   absorption by intestine—Maintains normal serum calcium and
   phosphorus levels
   Mobilizes phosphorus from soft tissues
   Mobilizes calcium from bone in hypocalcemia (with PTH)
   Converts organic phosphates to inorganic phosphates
   Catabolic

9. **Catabolism**
   Intermediates—Similar to cholesterol conversion products: bile acids and
      steroid hormones
   Excretion products
      No vit. D in urine (human)
      Animals—Excess vit. D into feces
      Humans—70% of ingested vit. D in feces as fecal sterols

MISCELLANEOUS

1. **Relationship to Other Vitamins**
   Vitamin A—
      Reduces toxic effects of vit. D
      Occurs naturally with vit. D in many fish oils
   Vitamin B_1—Increases tolerance of vit. D

2. **Relationship to Hormones**
   Parathormone—activity intensified by vit. D; deficiency of vit. D
      stimulates parathyroid
   Cortisone—Antagonizes effect of vit. D on citrate metabolism
   STH—A synergist in growth

3. **Unusual Features**
   Has hormonal qualities due to internal synthesis
   Vitamin D_2 little activity for chickens—species differ in response.
   May play role in aging calcification phenomena, especially in skin
   Can mimic rickets with high calcium low phosphorus diet
   Can mimic osteomalacia with low calcium high phosphorus diet
   Absorbed through skin
   Activates transport of heavy metals by intestinal cells
   Ample available for adults from most diets and skin synthesis
   Long acting, stored
   Furred and feathered animals obtain vit. D in grooming and licking
   Fish thought to obtain vit. D from marine invertebrates
   Useful in lead poisoning treatment

4. **Possible Relationships of Deficiency Symptoms to Metabolic Action**
   Decreased growth—Retarded calcification and bone growth
   Increased alkaline phosphatase—Attempt by organism to increase
      inorganic phosphate
   Osteomalacia—Demineralization of bone, (e.g. in pregnancy)
   Skeletal malformation—Retarded calcification

5
Vitamin E

GENERAL INFORMATION

1. **Synonyms:** α-Tocopherol, antisterility vitamin, 5,7,8,-trimethyltocol, Epsilan, Ephynal, Tokopharm, factor X

2. **History**
   - 1922—Evans and Bishop reported dietary factor "X" needed for normal rat reproduction
   - 1922—Matill found dietary factor "X" in yeast or lettuce
   - 1923—Evans *et al.* found factor "X" in alfalfa, wheat, oats, meat, butterfat
   - 1924—Sure named factor "X" vit. E.
   - 1936—Evans *et al.* demonstrated vit. E belongs to tocopherol family of compounds—isolated several active tocopherols—vit. E (α-tocopherol) most active of tocopherols
   - 1938—Fernholz determined structure of vit. E
   - 1938—Karrer synthesized vit. E
   - 1956—Green discovered eighth tocopherol

3. **Physiological Forms**
   d-α-tocopherol, tocopheronolactone, and their phosphate esters

4. **Active Analogs and Related Compounds**
   dl-α-Tocopherol, l-α-tocopherol, esters (succinate, acetate, phosphate), β, ζ_1, ζ_2-tocopherols

5. **Inactive Analogs and Related Compounds:** δ, ϵ, η-tocopherols

6. **Antagonists:** α-tocopherol quinone, oxidants, cod liver oil, thyroxine

7. **Synergists:** Vitamins A, B_6, B_{12}, C, K, folic acid, estradiol, testosterone, STH

8. **Physiological Functions**
   Biological antioxidant
   Normal growth maintenance
   Protects unsaturated fatty acids and membrane structures
   Aids intestinal absorption of unsaturated fatty acids
   Maintains normal muscle metabolism
   Maintains integrity of vascular system and central nervous system
   Detoxifying agent
   Maintenance of kidney tubules, lungs, genital structures, liver and RBC
      membranes

9. **Deficiency Diseases and Disorders**
   Laboratory animals—Degeneration of reproductive tissues, muscular
      dystrophy, encephalomalacia, liver necrosis
   Man—Skin collagenosis, red cell hemolysis, xanthomatosis, cirrhosis of
      gall bladder, steatorrhea, creatinuria

10. **Sources for Species Requiring It**
    Required by most organisms
       Exogenous sources—Man and higher vertebrates, protozoa, some
          microorganisms
       Endogenous sources—Plants, some microorganisms

CHEMISTRY

1. **Structure**

Vitamin E, $C_{29}H_{50}O_2$

2. **Reactions**

    Heat—Labile   Oxidation—Labile

    Acid—Stable   Reduction—Stable

    Alkali—Labile   Light—Labile (esp. UV)

    Water—Insol.

3. **Properties**

    Appearance—Yellow oil   Solubility

    MW—430.7 H_2O—Insol.

    MP—2.5-3.5°C   Acet., Alc.—Sol.

    Crystal Form—No data   Benz., Chl., Eth.—Sol.

    Salts, Esters—Succinate,   Absn. Max.—292 mμ (alc.)

      acetate, phosphate   Chemical Nature: Aromatic quinoid,

    Important Groups for activity   alc.

      Hydroxyl (alcoholic) $\alpha_D{}^{25} = +0.32°$ (alc.)

4. **Commercial Production:**   Molecular distillation from vegetable oils

5. **Isolation**

    Sources—Wheat germ oil, soybean oil, rice oil

    Method

      Saponify oil with methanolic KOH

      Nonsaponifiable fraction has vit. E, dissolve in ether

      Remove sterols with digitonin precipitation

      Remove xanthophylls with methanol extraction

      Convert tocopherols to allophanate esters with HCN

      Crystallize allophanates, hydrolyze, extract vit. E with ether

6. **Determination**

    Bioassay

      Rats—Prevent fetal resorption and RBC hemolysis

      Chick—Liver storage

    Physicochemical—Colorimetric 2-dimensional paper chromatography

DISTRIBUTION AND SOURCES

1. **Occurrence**

    Plants

      Fruit—Apples, olives

Vegetables—Legumes, lettuce, spinach, corn, soybean (oil), mustard, cauliflower, green peppers, turnip greens, kale, kohlrabi, sweet potatoes

Nuts and Seeds—Coconuts, peanuts, palm (oil), cottonseed

Grains—Cereals, oils (rice, wheat) oats, brown rice, wheat germ, barley, rye

Animals

Birds—Eggs

Mammals—Liver, fat, muscle, milk, pituitary, adrenals, testes

Microorganisms: Yeast

2. Dietary Sources

High: 50-300 mg/100 g

Oil (cottonseed, corn, soybean, safflower, wheat germ)

Margarine

Medium: 5-50 mg/100 g

Oils (coconut, peanut, olive)

Wheat germ, apple seeds, alfalfa, barley, dry soybeans, peanuts

Chocolate, rose hips, yeast

Cabbage, spinach, asparagus

Low: 0.5-5 mg/100 g

Brussel sprouts, carrots, parsnips, mustard, corn, brown rice, lettuce, cauliflower, peas, sweet potatoes, turnip greens, kale, kohlrabi, green peppers

Bacon, beef, lamb, pork, veal, beef liver

Eggs, butter, cheese

Whole wheat flour, dried navy beans, corn meal, oatmeal, coconut, rye, oats, wheat

Blackberries, pears, apples, olives

MEDICAL AND NUTRITIONAL ROLE

1. Units:

1 mg d-α-tocopherol = 1.49 I.U.

1 mg dl-α-tocopherol acetate = 1 I.U.

2. Normal Blood Levels (Man):   1.11 mg/100 ml (serum)

3. Recommended Allowances

Children—10-15 I.U./day

Adults—25 I.U./day (females); 30 I.U./day (males)

Special—Related to unsaturated fatty acid intake; increased requirements in pregnancy and lactation, detoxification, aging, stress

4. **Administration**
   Injection—No data
   Topical—No data
   Oral—Preferred route

5. **Factors Affecting Availability**
   Decrease
   Presence of antagonists
   Mineral oil ingestion
   Presence of vit. E oxidation products
   Occurrence with other less active analogues
   Excretion in feces
   Impaired fat absorption
   Chemical binding in foods
   Increased destruction (stress)
   Cooking losses—Heat and O_2 labile
   Losses in frozen storage, steatorrhea, variability of natural sources
   Increase
   Storage in (adipose and muscle) tissue
   Esterification increases stability
   Use of unprocessed fresh food sources
   Absorption aids—Bile salts

6. **Deficiency Symptoms**
   General
   RBC hemolysis
   Creatinuria
   Xanthomatosis and cirrhosis of gall bladder
   Steatorrhea (young)
   Cystic fibrosis of pancreas (young)
   Poorly developed muscles
   Muscular dystrophy (rats, dogs, monkeys, chickens)
   Myocardial degeneration (dogs, rabbits)
   Resorption of fetus, degeneration of germ epithelium, disturbance of estrus cycle (rats)
   Hepatic necrosis (rats)
   Encephalomalacia (chickens)
   Vascular degeneration (chickens)

7. **Effects of Overdose:**   Possible increase in blood pressure

METABOLIC ROLE

1. **Biosynthesis**
   Precursors—Mevalonic acid—Side chain (?); phenylalanine—ring (?)
   Intermediates—Tocotrienol

2. **Production:**   Species and Sites
   Plants—Nuts, seeds, cereal germ, green leaves, legumes
   Fungi—Yeast
   Bacteria—Various

3. **Storage Sites**
   Muscle—Small amounts
   Adipose tissues—Small amounts

4. **Blood Carriers:**   Lipoproteins

5. **Half-life:**   60-70% of daily dose ingested is excreted in feces

6. **Target Tissues:**   Kidneys, genital organs, muscles, liver, lungs, bone marrow

7. **Reactions**

Organ	Enzyme System

Muscle	Dehydrogenase
	    Xanthine oxidase
	    Isocitric dehydrogenase

Muscle	Protease—Cathepsin

Muscle	Phosphatase
	    Ribonuclease
	    Nucleotidase

Muscle	Glycosidase—glucuronidase

Muscle	Miscellaneous
	    Creatine kinase
	    Cytochrome c reductase

8. Mode of Action

Cellular

Anabolic—Maintains protein synthesis by prevention of formation of enzyme-toxic peroxides from unsaturated fatty acid

Catabolic—Participates in oxidation-reduction reactions via CoQ and respiratory enzyme systems

Other—Protects unsaturated fatty acids against oxidation; maintains structure of cellular, mitochondrial, microsomal, and lysosomal membranes

Organismal

Anabolic—increases N retention

Maintains kidney tubules and genital organs

Maintains muscle cell membranes

9. Catabolism

Intermediates—tocopheryl-*p*-quinone

Excretion products

Breath—CO_2

Urine—Water soluble degradation products, tocopheronic acid glucuronate, tocopheronolactone glucuronate

MISCELLANEOUS

1. Relationship to Other Vitamins

Vitamin C—Reduces oxidized vit. E back to vit. E in rats

Decreased synthesis of vit. C in vit. E deficient animals

Vitamin A—Conserved by vit. E in chick; protected against oxidation by vit. E; synergizes with vit. E in promoting growth and disease resistance

Vitamin B_{12} and Folic Acid

Act with vit. E in treatment of macrocytic anemia

Vit. E can substitute for or potentiate vit. B_{12}

Vitamin K and CoQ

Very similar in structure to vit. E

Pantothenic acid—Promotes synthesis of vit. E in plants

2. Relationship to Hormones

> FSH and LH—Production increased in vit. E deficiency
>
> Testosterone—Testicular degeneration due to vit. E deficiency in rats causes decreased production of testosterone
>
> High content of vit. E in testicular tissues, seminal fluid
>
> Cortisone—Requirements for cortisone and vit. E increase during stress. High content of vit. E at sites of cortisone synthesis in adrenal cortex
>
> STH—A synergist in growth

3. Unusual Features

> May be involved in aging mechanisms by protecting unsaturated fatty acids and membranes against free radicals
>
> Only d-isomers occur naturally
>
> Vitamin E replaceable by selenium salts in therapy of rat and pig liver necrosis, and chick exudative diathesis
>
> Vitamin E replaceable by CoQ and antioxidants for certain symptoms of vit. E deficiency but not for all, e.g., RBC hemolysis, resorption gestation not affected.
>
> Species differences in response to vit. E treatment of similar symptoms, e.g. muscular dystrophy—rabbits positive, humans negative
>
> Other tocopherols only slightly active compared to vit. E
>
> Decreased in tumors

4. Possible Relationships of Deficiency Symptoms to Metabolic Action

> Muscular dystrophy, creatinuria (rabbit, monkey)—Maintenance of muscle cell membranes
>
> RBC hemolysis (man)—Maintenance of red cell membranes
>
> Fetal resorption (rats)—Maintenance of uterine membranes and uterine nerve ganglia
>
> Mycardial degeneration (dog, rabbit)—Maintenance of muscle cell membranes

Steatorrhea (man)—Impaired lipid absorption by intestinal cells; maintenance of intestinal cell membranes

Encephalomalacia (chick)—Maintenance of nerve and membrane structures

6
Vitamin K

GENERAL INFORMATION

1. **Synonyms:**   Antihemorrhagic vitamin, prothrombin factor, Koagulations-vitamin

2. **History**
   1929—Dam reported chicks on synthetic diet develop hemorrhagic conditions
   1935—Dam named vit. K as the missing factor in synthetic diet
   1935—Almquist and Stokstad demonstrated vit. K present in fish meal and alfalfa
   1939—Dam and Karrer isolated vit. K from alfalfa
   1939—Doisy isolated K_1 from alfalfa, K_2 from fish meal, and demonstrated difference
   1939—MacCorquodale, Cheney, Fieser determined structure of vit. K_1
   1939—Almquist and Klose synthesized vit. K_1
   1941—Link *et al.* discovered dicoumarol

3. **Physiological Forms**
   Plant—Vitamin K_1 (phylloquinone, phytonadione)
   Animal—Vitamin $K_{2(20)}$.
   Bacterial—Vitamin K_2 (farnoquinone) ($K_{2(30)}$, $K_{2(35)}$)

4. **Active Analogs and Related Compounds**
   Menadiol diphosphate, menadione (vit. K_3), menadione bisulfite
   Phthiocol, synkayvite, menadiol (vit. K_4), vits. K_5, K_6, K_7

5. **Inactive Analogs and Related Compounds:**   Reduced vit. K

6. **Antagonists:**   Dicoumarol,   sulfonamides,   antibiotics,   α-tocopherol quinone, dihydroxystearic acid glycide, salicylates, iodinin, warfarin

7. **Synergists:**   Vitamins E, A, C; STH

8. **Physiological Functions:**   Prothrombin synthesis in liver, blood-clotting mechanisms,   electron   transport   mechanisms,   growth,   photosynthetic mechanisms

9. **Deficiency Diseases, Disorders:**   Hypoprothrombinemia

10. **Sources for Species Requiring It:**
    Many species require it
    Exogenous sources: Vertebrates, some bacteria. (Intestinal bacteria provide in man)
    Endogenous sources: Plants, bacteria, and all other organisms requiring it

CHEMISTRY

1. **Structure**

Vitamin K_1, $C_{31}H_{46}O_2$

2. **Reactions**

Heat—Stable	Oxidation—Stable
Acid—(Strong) labile	Reduction—Labile
Alkali—Labile	Light—Labile
Water—Insol.	

3. **Properties**

Appearance—Yellow oil	Important Groups for activity
MW—450.7	Menadiol nucleus
MP— −20°C	Phytyl side chain
Crystal Form—No data	*Trans*-methyl groups
Salts—Disodium phosphate	

Solubility   Absn. Max.—243, 249, 260,
  H_2O—Insol.   269, 325 mμ (hexane)
  Acet., Alc.—Sol.   Chemical Nature: Quinone
  Benz. Chl. Eth.—Sol. $\alpha_D^{20} = -0.4°C$ (benzene)

4. Commercial Production: Column Chromatography of fish meal extracts

5. Isolation
   Sources—Fish meal, alfalfa
   Method
      Remove chlorophyll from pet. ether extract by column chroma-
         tography on $ZnCO_3$
      Reduce to hydroquinone using sodium hydrosulfite
      Extract with pet. ether, alkali, ether
      Oxidize hydroquinone to quinone

6. Determination
   Bioassay—Vitamin K deficient chick assay
   Physicochemical—Polarographic methods; spectrophotometry of pure
      solutions; prothrombin time determination

DISTRIBUTION AND SOURCES

1. Occurrence
   Plants:
      Fruit—Orange (peel), tomato
      Vegetables—Spinach, cabbage, brussel sprouts, alfalfa, cauliflower,
         soybean (oil)
      Nuts and seeds—Hemp seed
   Animals: Pork liver, eggs, milk, fish meal
   Microorganisms: Intestinal bacteria, *M. phlei*

2. Dietary Sources
   High: 100-300 μg/100 g
      Cabbage, cauliflower, soybeans, spinach
      Pork, Beef liver, beef kidney
   Medium: 10-100 μg/100 g
      Potatoes, strawberries, tomatoes, alfalfa, wheat (whole, germ, bran),
         pine needles, egg yolk
   Low: 0-10 μg/100 g
      Corn, carrots, peas, parsley, mushrooms, milk

MEDICAL AND NUTRITIONAL ROLE

1. **Units:**   0.0008 mg menadione = 20 dam units = 1 ansbacher unit

2. **Normal Blood Levels (Man):**   Not reported

3. **Recommended Allowances**
   Children—Supplied by intestinal bacteria normally
   Adults—Supplied by intestinal bacteria normally
   Special
       Increases with external temperature
       Newborn infants with neonatal hemorrhage
       Mothers in labor
       Overdosage with anticoagulants

4. **Administration**
   Injection—Intravenous, intramuscular
   Topical—No data
   Oral—Occasionally

5. **Factors Affecting Availability**
   Decrease
       Biliary obstruction
       Liver damage—cirrhosis, toxins
       Poor food preparation conditions
       Presence of antagonists
       Impaired lipid absorption in gut
       Ingestion of mineral oil
       Sterilization of gut with antibiotics and sulfa drugs
       Excretion in feces
   Increase
       Storage in liver
       Absorption aids—bile salts

6. **Deficiency Symptoms**
   Hypoprothrombinemia—General
   Increased bleeding and hemorrhage—General
   Increased clotting time—General
   Neonatal hemorrhage—General
   Internal hemorrhage (chick)

7. Effects of Overdose
    Usually nontoxic, occasionally toxic
    Possible thrombosis, vomiting, porphyrinuria—man
    Albuminuria—dog
    Increased clotting time—rabbit
    Cytopenia, hemoglobinemia—mouse
    Kernicterus (menadione)

METABOLIC ROLE

1. Biosynthesis
    Precursors—Polyacetic acid (ring); acetate (side chain)
    Intermediates—Dehydroquinic acid (ring); farnesol (side chain)

2. Production: Species and sites
    Plants—green leaves
    Bacteria—intestinal (main source)

3. Storage Sites: Liver (small)

4. Blood Carriers: Lipoproteins

5. Half-life: Depletion causes deficiency within 10 days in rat

6. Target tissues: Liver, vascular system

7. Reactions
    Coenzyme form—Vitamin $K_{2(20)}$, CoQ(?)

Organ	Enzyme System	Effect
	Electron transport	
Bacteria	Malate reductase	Activated
Bacteria	DPNH dehydrogenase	Activated
Liver	Vit. K reductase	Reduction of vit. K
Liver	Oxidative phosphorylation	Completes system
Liver	Respiratory chain	Completes system

8. **Mode of Action**

    Cellular

        Anabolic

            Prothrombin synthesis (liver)

            β-Globulin synthesis (liver)

            Photosynthesis-Hill reaction

        Catabolic—Decreases phosphate incorporation into liver RNA

        Other—Mitochondrial electron transport systems component

    Organismal

        Maintenance of prothrombin and clotting factors VII, IX, X

        Control internal hemorrhage

        Anabolic—Increase nitrogen retention

9. **Catabolism**

    Intermediates—Lactones

    Excretion products—As glucuronide and sulfate conjugates in urine, bile, feces

MISCELLANEOUS

1. **Relationship to Other Vitamins**

    Vitamin E—Synergistic to vit. K—Maintains reduced state similar in structure to vit. K_1 and probably interconvertible by way of CoQ and ubichromenols

    Vitamins A and C—Fragility of RBC correlated with vits. A, C, K

2. **Relationship to Hormones**

    STH—Synergist in growth

3. **Unusual Features**

    Intestinal absorption of vit. K in chicks poor

    Side chains of vit. K identical to those in ubiquinones (CoQ)

    Completely supplied by intestinal flora in normal adults

    Vitamin K lost on γ-irradiation of foods

4. **Possible Relationships of Deficiency Symptoms to Metabolic Action**

    Hemorrhage—Decreased synthesis of prothrombin and other clotting factors by the liver

7
Thiamine

GENERAL INFORMATION

1. Synonyms: Vitamin B_1, aneurin, antineuritic factor, antiberiberi factor, oryzamin

2. History

1897—Eijkman ameliorated beriberi in humans by addition of rice polishings to diet

1911—Funk isolated dietary growth factor from rice polishings which cured beriberi; coined term "vitamine"

1915—McCollum and Davis proposed term "water-soluble B" for antiberiberi factor

1920—Emmet and Luros demonstrated two growth factors in rice polishings, including antiberiberi factor destroyed by autoclaving

1926—Jansen and Donath isolated crystalline antiberiberi factor from rice bran

1927—Brit. Med. Res. Council proposed name of B_1 for antiberiberi factor

1936—Williams synthesized B_1 and named it thiamine

3. Physiological Forms

Thiamine pyrophosphate (cocarboxylase)—Animals

Thiamine orthophosphate—Animals

Free thiamine—Plants

4. **Active Analogs and Related Compounds**
   Ethyl substituted for methyl on pyrimidine C-2
   Thiamine disulfide, acylated thiamine

5. **Inactive Analogs and Related Compounds:**   Reduced thiamine

6. **Antagonists:**   Pyrithiamine, oxythiamine, 2-*n*-butyl homologue

7. **Synergists:**   Vitamins B_{12}, B_2, B_6, niacin, pantothenic acid, STH

8. **Physiological Functions:**   Coenzyme in pyruvate metabolism; growth, appetite, digestion, nerve activity, gastrointestinal tonus, carbohydrate metabolism, energy production

9. **Deficiency Diseases, Disorders:**   Beriberi, opisthotonos (in birds), polyneuritis, hyperesthesia, bradycardia, edema

10. **Sources for Species Requiring It**
    All species require it for life
    Exogenous sources—All animals, some (algae, fungi, bacteria). Not much available from intestinal bacteria in man, although it is made there
    Endogenous sources—Some (algae, fungi, bacteria), all higher plants. Sheep and cattle get sufficiency from intestinal bacteria

CHEMISTRY

1. **Structure**

Pyrimidine   Thiazole

Thiamine hydrochloride,
$C_{12}H_{17}N_4OSCl \cdot HCl$

2. **Reactions**

Heat—Labile	Oxidation—Forms thiochrome
Acid—Stable	(fluoresc.)
Alkali—Unstable	Reduction—Unstable
Water—Acid (HCl)	Light—UV decomposes

3. **Properties**

Appearance—White
crystals
MW—337.3 (as HCl)
MP—244°C
Crystal Form—
Monocl. plates
Salts—Mononitrate,
noble metals
Important Groups for activity
—OH of —CH_2CH_2OH
C-2 of pyrimidine
C-2 of thiazole

Solubility
H_2O—1 g/ml H_2O
Alc.—sol.
Acet. Benz., Chl., Eth.—Insol
Absn. Max.—235, 267 mμ
Chemical Nature—Base, alc.,
substituted pyrimidine
Misc.—Charact. odor
pKa = 4.8, 9.2
α_D = 0 (inactive)

4. **Commercial Production:**   Synthesis

Pyrimidine + thiazole nuclei synthesized separately and then condensed
Build on pyrimidine with acetamidine

5. **Isolation**

Sources—Rice bran, wheat germ, yeast
Method—Aqueous extraction, adsorption on Fuller's earth; elute with
quinine sulfate, precipitate as phosphotungstate, decompose precipitate and reprecipitate with $AuCl_3$, extract with water, precipitate from EtOH as hydrochloride

6. **Determination**

Bioassay—Yeast fermentation; polyneuritic rat—rate of cure; bacterial
metabolism
Physicochemical—Thiochrome fluorescence; polarographic; chromatographic; absorption at 235-267 mμ in neutral solution; at 247 in
acid solution

DISTRIBUTION AND SOURCES

1. **Occurrence**

Plants

Fruit—All. Low (except gooseberries, plums, which are medium)
Vegetables—All. Low (except beans, green leafy types, cauliflower,
corn, peas, potatoes—medium)
Nuts—All. Medium (except coconut, which is low)
Grains—All. Medium (except outer grain kernels, bran, polishings,
wheat germ, which are high)

Animals: All—Medium (except pork, which is high, and some fish, which are low)

Microorganisms: Yeast (killed)—high. Intestinal bacteria not available

Misc.—Mushrooms—medium

2. **Dietary Sources**

High: 1000-10,000 μg/100 g

Wheat germ, rice bran, soybean flour

Yeast

Ham

Medium: 100-1000 μg/100 g

Gooseberries, plums, prunes (dry), raisins (dry), asparagus, beans (kidney, lima, snap, soy, wax), beet greens, broccoli, brussel sprouts, cauliflower, chicory, endive, corn, dandelion greens, kale, kohlrabi, leeks, lentils (dry), parsley, peas, potatoes, watercress, barley, oats, rice (brown), almonds, brazil, cashews, chestnuts, hazelnuts, peanuts, pecans, walnuts

Beef, calf, chicken, pork, lamb, turkey meat and organs, mushrooms

Eggs, milk, carp, clams, cod, lobster, mackerel, oysters, salmon

Low: 10-100 μg/100 g

Apples, apricots, avocados, bananas, berries (black-, blue-, cran-, rasp-, straw-), melons (cantaloupe, water, honeydew), cherries, currants, dates (dry), figs, grapes, grapefruit, lemons, oranges, peaches, pears, pineapples, prunes, tangerines

Artichokes, beets, cabbage, carrots, celery, cucumbers, eggplant, lettuce, onions, parsnips, peppers, pumpkins, radishes, rhubarb, spinach, sweet potatoes, turnips, coconut, cheeses, flounder

Haddock, halibut, herring, pike, sardines, scallops, shrimp, trout, tuna

MEDICAL AND NUTRITIONAL ROLE

1. **Units:** 1 USP unit = 3 μg thiamine HCl = 1 I.U.

2. **Normal Blood Levels (Man):** 1.3 μg/100 free base in serum. 3-11 μg/100 cocarboxylase in blood cells

3. **Recommended Allowances**

Children—0.6-1.1 mg/day

Adults—1.0 mg/day, female; 1.4 mg/day, male

Special—Increased requirements in pregnancy and lactation. Depends on body weight, calorie intake, intestinal synthesis and absorption, fat content of diet (increased pyruvate)

4. Administration

    Injection—Intravenous, intraperitoneal

    Topical—No data

    Oral—Preferred route

5. Factors Affecting Availability

    Decrease

        Cooking—heat labile, water soluble

        Enzymes in food; thiaminase for vitamin breakdown

        Destruction by $CaCO_3$, K_2HPO_4, $MnSO_4$

        Nitrites, sulfites destroy

        Diuresis, gastrointestinal diseases

        Live yeast, alkali

    Increase

        Cellulose in diet increases intestinal synthesis

        Small storage capacity in heart, liver, kidney

        Bacterial synthesis in intestine (normally none)

6. Deficiency Symptoms

    General (Man); beriberi

        Anesthesia, hyperesthesia

        Retarded growth, neuron degeneration

        Fatigue, weight loss, anorexia, G.I. complaints, weakness, loss of reflexes, and vibratory sense

        Circulatory and cardiac involvement

        Mental disturbances—depression, irritability, memory loss

        Muscular atrophy in extremities

        Increased blood pyruvate and lactate

    Lab animals

        Decreased fat stores, decreased body temperature

        Neurological disturbance—polyneuritis, decrease in tone

        Bradycardia, cardiac enlargement, edema

        Opisthotonos (chickens, pigeons, turkey)

7. Effects of Overdose

    Humans—Limited toxicity, starting at approx. 125-350 mg/kg dosage. Edema, nervousness, sweating, tachycardia, tremors, herpes, allergicity, fatty liver, vascular hypotension

    Rats—Sterility, B_6 Deficiency

METABOLIC ROLE

1. **Biosynthesis**
   Precursors—Thiazole, pyrimidine pyrophosphate
   Intermediates—Thiamine phosphate

2. **Production Sites**
   Plants—Grain and cereal germ
   Bacteria—Intestinal

3. **Storage Sites:** Heart, liver, kidney, brain (all small amounts)

4. **Blood Carriers:** Blood cells—As cocarboxylase. Serum—free B_1

5. **Half-life:** 1 mg/day destroyed in tissues

6. **Target Tissues:** Heart, liver, kidney, peripheral nerves, brain

7. **Reactions**
   Coenzyme Forms—cocarboxylase (thiamine pyrophosphate, disphospho-thiamine). Needs Mg^{++} ion

Organ	Enzyme System	Effect
Liver, plants	Transketolase	Activated
Serum	Choline esterase	Inhibited
Liver, yeast	Thiaminokinase—thiamine → cocarboxylase	Activated

Plants	Decarboxylases:
	    Nonoxidate decarboxylation of pyruvate
	    to OAA
		Activated

Liver (mammals)	Oxidative decarboxylation of pyruvate with lipoic acid	Activated
Liver (mammals)	Phosphoroclastic cleavage of α-keto acids	Activated
Liver (mammals)	Formation of acetoin	Activated
Liver (mammals)	Oxidative decarboxylation of α-ketoglutarate to succinate	Activated

8. **Mode of Action**
   Cellular
      Anabolic—Condensations, synthesis of acetylcholine
      Catabolic—α-Keto acid decarboxylation (Krebs cycle coenzyme—ATP generation), oxidations, dismutations
      Other—Transketolation, formation of NADPH, and ribose via HMP shunt, acyl transfer agent—"active" acetaldehyde

Organismal
   Maintenance of nerve tissues
   Maintenance of heart muscle
   Decrease blood pyruvate and lactate
   Maintain supply of ATP
   Normal growth maintenance

9. **Catabolism:**   Intermediates—Pyrimidine.   Excretion   products—Pyrimidine
   and thiamine

MISCELLANEOUS

1. **Relationship to Other Vitamins**
   Vitamin B_{12}—Synergistic to B_1
   Pantothenic Acid, Niacin, Riboflavin—Energy from oxidation of carbo-
      hydrates depends on synergism with thiamine (oxidative decarboxy-
      lation)
   Vitamin C—Decreases requirement for B_1
   Vitamin B_6—Overdose of B_1 causes B_6 deficiency in rats
   Vitamin D—Tolerance increased by vit. B_1
   Riboflavin, Pyridoxine—Synergize with thiamine to produce niacin

2. **Relationship to Hormones**
   Acetylcholine—Synthesis requires vit. B_1
   Thyroxine—Metabolic rate increase in hyperthyroidism increases B_1
      requirement
   Insulin—In diabetes B_1 content of blood and liver reduced
   STH—Synergist in growth

3. **Unusual features**
   Hormonal function in plants—controls root growth
   Phosphorylation in liver, dephosphorylation in kidney
   Vitamin B enzymes easily poisoned by heavy metals, mustard gas, acetyl
      iodide
   Plant and animal cocarboxylases identical
   Has a diuretic effect, is constipative
   Can be allergenic on injection
   Blood contains most cocarboxylase in leukocytes
   Thiamine sparing action by alcohol, fat, protein
   Not available from intestinal bacteria

4. Possible Relationships of Deficiency to Metabolic Action

Flooding of system with pyruvate

Weight loss

G.I. complaints

Fatigue

Anorexia

Decreased synthesis of acetylcholine

Polyneuritis

Mental disturbances

Circulatory and cardiac involvement

8
Riboflavin

GENERAL INFORMATION

1. **Synonyms:** Vitamin B_2, vit. G, lactoflavin, hepatoflavin, ovoflavin, verdo-
   flavin, 6,7-dimethyl-9-(d-1'-ribityl)isoalloxazine

2. **History**
   1917—Emmet and McKim showed dietary growth factor for rats in rice
   polishings
   1920—Emmett suggested presence of several dietary growth factors in
   yeast concentrate, including heat-stable component and B_1
   1927—Brit. Med. Res. Council proposed name of B_2 for heat-stable
   component
   1932—Warburg and Christian isolated yellow enzyme (containing riboflavin (FMN)) from bottom yeast
   1933—Kuhn isolated pure B_2 (riboflavin) from milk; recognized growth
   promoting activity
   1935—Kuhn *et al.*; Karrer *et al.*—Achieved structure and synthesis of vit.
   B_2; named it riboflavin
   1954—Christie *et al.* determined structure and synthesized FAD

3. **Physiological Forms:** Riboflavin mononucleotide (FMN). Riboflavin dinucleotide (FAD)

4. **Active Analogs and Related Compounds:** 7-Methyl-9-methyl, and 6-ethyl-
   7-methyl compounds, arabinoflavin

5. **Inactive   Analogs   and   Related   Compounds:**   3,6,7-Trimethyl-
   9-(d-1'-ribityl)isoalloxazine

6. **Antagonists:** Isoriboflavin, lumiflavin, araboflavin, hydroxyethyl analogue,
   formyl methyl analogue, galactoflavin, flavin mono-SO_4

7. **Synergists:** Vitamins A, B_1, B_6, B_{12}, niacin, pantothenic acid, folic acid,
   biotin, T4, insulin, STH

8. **Physiological Functions**
   Coenzyme in respiratory enzyme systems
   Constituent of flavoproteins, redox systems, respiratory enzymes
   Growth and development of fetus
   Maintenance of mucosal, epithelial, and eye tissues

9. **Deficiency Diseases, Disorders:** Glossitis, cheilosis, seborrheic dermatitis,
   corneal vascularization, anemia

10. **Sources for Species Requiring It**
    All organisms require it
    Endogenous sources—Higher plants, algae, some bacteria, some fungi
    Exogenous sources—All animals, some fungi and bacteria (intestinal
    bacteria make it, but most is unavailable to man)

CHEMISTRY

1. **Structure**

Riboflavin, $C_{17}H_{20}O_6N_4$

Purine

2. Reactions

Heat—Blackens at 240°C

Acid—Stable

Alkali—Labile → lumiflavin

Water—Soluble, acidic

Oxidation—Decomposes

Reduction—Easily → leucoribo-
flavin

Light—Photolyses to lumiflavin
Intense green fluorescence
565 mµ

3. Properties

Appearance—Orange-yellow
powder

MW—376.4

MP—282°C

Crystal Form—Needles

Salts—Borate, PO$_4$, acetate

Important Groups
9-N, 5'-OH
6,7-methyl
3-N

Solubility

H$_2$O—Sol. 0.01 g/100 ml

Acet., Alc.—Insol.

Benz., Chl., Eth.—Insol.

Absn. Max.—220, 267, 336,
446 mµ

Misc.—pl = 6

$[\alpha]_D^{20} = -114°$ (0.1 N NaOH)

Chemical Nature

Reducing agent; nucleotide

Substituted purine

4. Commercial Production

Fermentation bacteria or yeast

Chemical synthesis from alloxan, ribose, and o-xylene

5. Isolation

Sources—Free—urine, whey, retina. Combined—as FMN or FAD—tissues
or egg whites

Method

Aq. extract of tissue treated with ether

Fractional pptn. with picric acid

Ppt. out proteins with ammon sulfate

Adsorb on Fuller's earth

Elute with 0.1 N NaOH

Crystallize from aq. pet. ether-acetone mixture

6. Determination

Bioassay—Rats—growth rate. Microbiological—*L caseii, L. mesenteroides*

Physicochemical—Fluorimetry, paper electrophoresis, polarography

DISTRIBUTION AND SOURCES

1. **Occurrence**
   Plants
     Fruit—All. Low
     Vegetables—All. High in tomato leaves. Medium in green leafy types, corn, cauliflower, beans. Low in others
     Nuts—All. Medium except coconut (low)
     Flowers—Saffron (high)
   Animals—All (liver > kidneys > heart > other tissues). High in organs, medium in other tissues. Crustaceans—High
   Microorganisms: All, esp. yeast, anerobic bacteria (high)

2. **Dietary Sources**
   High: 1000-10,000 μg/100 g
     Beef (kidneys, liver), calf (kidney, liver)
     Chicken (liver)
     Pork (heart, kidneys, liver), sheep (liver, kidneys)
     Yeast (killed)
   Medium: 100-1000 μg/100 g
     Avocados, currants
     Asparagus, beans (kidney, lima, snap, wax), beet greens, broccoli, brussel sprouts, cauliflower, chicory, endive, corn, dandelion greens, kale, kohlrabi, lentils (dry), parsley, parsnips, peas, soybeans (dry), spinach, turnip greens, watercress, almonds (dry), cashews, peanuts, pecans, walnuts, rice bran, wheat germ, oats, cheeses, cream, eggs, milk
     Bacon, beef, chicken, duck, goose, pork, lamb, turkey, veal, fish
   Low: 10-100 μg/100 g
     Apples, apricots, bananas, blackberries, blueberries, cranberries, raspberries, strawberries, cherries, grapes, grapefruit, melons, oranges, peaches, dates (dry), figs, pears, pineapples, plums, raisins (dry), tangerines, artichokes, beets, cabbages, carrots, celery, cucumbers, eggplant, lettuce, onions, peppers, potatoes, pumpkins, radishes, sweet potatoes, tomatoes, turnips, coconuts, barley, rice

MEDICAL AND NUTRITIONAL ROLE

1. **Units:** By weight, μg or mg

2. **Normal Blood Levels:** 6.6 μg/100 ml

3. **Recommended Allowances**
   Children—0.6-1.2 mg/day*
   Adults—1.5 mg/day female*; 1.7 mg/day male*

4. **Administration**
   Injection—I.V.
   Topical—No data
   Oral—Preferred route

5. **Factors Affecting Availability**
   Decrease
   Cooking (sl. sol. in H_2O)
   Plant foods—Lower availability, bound forms
   Decreased phosphorylation in intestines prevents absorption
   Exposure of foods to sunlight
   Enzymes for breakdown
   Gastrointestinal disease
   Diuresis
   Increase
   Storage in heart, liver and kidneys
   Very actively producing intestinal bacteria (small amount)

6. **Deficiency Symptoms**
   General
   Orogenital syndrome
   Stomatitis
   Glossitis
   Cheilosis
   Seborrheic dermatitis
   Ocular—Photophobia, indistinct vision, corneal vascularity increased
   Rats
   Poor growth, ocular abnormality
   Dermatitis (eczema—nostrils, eyes)
   Myelin degeneration, testicular atrophy
   Thymus involution
   Dogs
   Weight loss, fatty liver, muscle weakness
   Opacity of corneal epithelium

* Related to caloric intake and protein levels. Increased in pregnancy, lactation. Additional sources in intestinal bacteria (small).

Chicken
 Egg production and hatchability decline, nerve degeneration
Monkey
 Anemia, leukopenia

7. **Effects of Overdose**
 Essentially nontoxic in man
 Anuria—rat
 Azotemia—rat
 Kidney insufficiency—rat
 Paresthesia—man
 Itching—man

METABOLIC ROLE

1. **Biosynthesis**
 Precursors—Purines, pyrimidines, ribose
 Intermediates—6,7-Dimethyl-8-ribityllumazine

2. **Production Site**
 Plants—Leaves, germinating seeds, root nodules
 Bacteria—Intestinal

3. **Storage Sites:** Heart, liver, kidneys (small amount)

4. **Blood carriers:** As nucleotides

5. **Half-life:** 12% of intake excreted in 24 hr

6. **Target Tissues:** Heart, liver, kidneys, others in lesser amount

7. **Reactions**
 Coenzyme forms
  Redox couple: oxidized $\rightleftharpoons$ reduced form
  FMN, FAD (binding to apoenzyme via cations (Fe^{++}, Cu^{++}, Mo^{++}) to PO_4 of coenzyme)

Organ	Enzyme System	Effect
Liver	(1) FMN—Warburg yellow enzyme, cytochrome C reductase, l-amino acid, oxidase succinic dehydrogenase	Activated
Liver	(2) FAD—Xanthine oxidase, d-amino acid oxidase, glycine oxidase, diaphorase, fumaric dehydrogenase, glucose oxidases, histaminases, aldehyde oxidase	Activated
Intestine	(3) Flavokinase—Phosphorylation of riboflavin	Activated

8. **Mode of Action**
    Cellular
        Anabolic—No data
        Catabolic—Carbohydrate metabolism
        Other—Essential complexed part of flavoproteins
            Mitochondrial electron transport system
            Oxidation-reduction enzyme systems
            Accepts 2H on isoalloxazine ring
            Part of respiratory enzyme system
    Organismal
        Ectodermal maintenance—skin and cornea
        Growth and development of fetus
        Maintenance of nervous system (myelin sheath)
        Resistance to disease

9. **Catabolism**
    Intermediates—No data
    Excretion products
        Urine—Free vitamin—Diurnal variations. Normally ~1/3 of dietary amounts excreted
        Feces—Uroflavin—Diurnal variations

MISCELLANEOUS

1. **Relationship to Other Vitamins**
    Vitamin A, Niacin—Present with riboflavin in visual structures (retina) involved in visual process
    Niacin—Riboflavin enzymes utilize DPN, and DPNH
    Thiamine—Deficiency of B_1 leads to increased storage of riboflavin. Involved with riboflavin in thyroxine and insulin utilization in CHO metabolism
    Other B vitamins—Synergistic with riboflavin

2. Relationship to Hormones

ACTH—Riboflavin involved in release of ACTH from pituitary

Thyroxine, Insulin—Effective only if riboflavin and thiamine are present

Thyroxine—Incorporation of iodide by sheep thyroid stimulated by FMN

Adrenal hormones—Aid in phosphorylation of riboflavin in intestines

Estradiol—Inactivation in liver decreased in riboflavin deficiency (rat)

STH—Synergist in growth

3. Unusual Features

High levels in liver inhibit tumor formation by azo compounds in animals

Free radicals formed by light or dehydrogenation: flavine $\rightleftharpoons$ semi-quinone $\rightleftharpoons$ dihydroflavin

Free vitamin only in retina, urine, milk and semen

Substitution of adenine by other purines, pyrimidines destroys activity of FAD

Phosphorylation of vitamin in intestines allows absorption as FMN

Blood levels decrease during life in humans

Brain content remains constant

Available in plants as FMN and FAD

Concentrated in bull semen

4. Possible Relationships of Deficiency Symptoms to Metabolic Action

Ectodermal manifestations related to other B-vitamin deficiencies

Cheilosis

Glossitis

Stomatitis

Seborrheic dermatitis

Corneal vascularity

Orogenital syndrome

Synergistic functions of vit. A and riboflavin in visual structures—Photophobia

9
Vitamin B$_6$

GENERAL INFORMATION

1. **Synonyms:** Pyridoxine, adermine, pyridoxol

2. **History**
   - 1934—György cured a dermatitis in rats not due to B$_1$ or B$_2$ with yeast extract factor
   - 1938—Lepkovsky isolated similar factor from rice bran extract
   - 1938—Keresztesy and Stevens isolated and crystallized pure B$_6$ from rice polishings
   - 1938—Kohn, Wendt, and Westphal synthesized pyridoxine, gave pyridoxine its name
   - 1939—Stiller, Keresztesy, and Stevens established structure of pyridoxine
   - 1945—Snell discovered pyridoxal and pyridoxamine
   - 1953—Snyderman *et al.* first recognized and established B$_6$ requirement in humans

3. **Physiological Forms**
   Interconvertible *in vivo* (pyridoxine $\rightleftharpoons$ pyridoxal $\rightleftharpoons$ pyridoxamine)
   Animals—Pyridoxal-5-phosphate (codecarboxylase); pyridoxamine phosphate
   Plants—Pyridoxol-5-phosphate, pyridoxal-5-P, pyridoxamine-P

4. **Active Analogs and Related Compounds:** Pyridoxal, pyridoxamine

5. **Inactive Analogs and Related Compounds:** Nor-vitamin B$_6$, 4-pyridoxic acid, 5-pyridoxic acid

6. **Antagonists:** 4-deoxypyridoxine, 4-methoxypyridoxine, toxopyrimidine, penicillamine, semicarbazide, isoniazid

7. **Synergists:** Vitamins B$_1$, B$_2$, C, E, niacin, biotin, folic acid, STH, glucagon, epinephrine, norepinephrine

8. **Physiological Functions**
   Protein, CHO, and lipid metabolism
   Coenzyme in many phases of amino acid metabolism; especially in gluconeogenesis, production of neural hormones, bile acids, unsaturated fatty acids, and porphyrins
   Erythrocyte formation, growth

9. **Deficiency Diseases, Disorders**
   Monkey—Arteriosclerosis
   Rats—Acrodynia
   Man—Lymphopenia, convulsions, dermatitis, irritability, nervous disorders

10. **Sources for Species Requiring It**
    All animals require B$_6$
    Exogenous sources—Animals, some bacteria (intestinal bacteria make it, but not much is available to man)
    Endogenous sources—Plants, fungi, intestinal bacteria

CHEMISTRY

1. **Structures**

Pyridoxine, C$_8$H$_{11}$NO$_3$ Pyridoxal   Pyridoxamine

2. Reactions

Heat—Stable

Acid—Stable

Alkali—Stable

Water—Basic

Oxidation—Unstable

Reduction—Unstable

Light—Labile (stable in acid)

3. Properties

Appearance—White powder

MW—169 pyridoxine

MP—160° pyridoxine

Crystal Form—Platelets

Salts—Hydrochloride, Ca^{++}

Important Groups for activity

$-CH_2OH$

$-N=$

Solubility

H_2O—0.2 g/ml

Acet., Alc.—Sol.

Benz., Chl., Eth.—Insol.

Absn. Max.—256, 327 mµ

pH 7.0

Chemical Nature

hydroxylated weak nitrogen base, substituted pyridine

pKa = 5.0, 8.9

αD = 0 (inactive)

4. Commercial Production

Commercially available as pyridoxine hydrochloride

Synthesized by method of Harris and Folkers. Ethoxy acetylacetone condensed with cyanoacetamide

Easiest route for synthesis is probably from oxazoles

5. Isolation

Sources—Rice polishings or bran and yeast

Methods

Adsorption on Fuller's earth or charcoal

Elute with $Ba(OH)_2$

Precipitate impurities with heavy metals

Precipitation with phosphotungstic acid

6. Determination

Bioassay—Animal

Rat acrodynia test

Rat growth and chicken growth assays

Tryptophane loading test

Blood cell

Bioassay—Microbial—Microbioassay

Physicochemical—Photofluorometric procedure detects 4-pyridoxic acid- (major metabolite) in urine. Chromatographic procedure to detect 4-pyridoxic acid

DISTRIBUTION AND SOURCES

1. **Occurrence**
   Plants
   Fruit—All low, except bananas, avocados, grapes, pears (medium)
   Vegetables—All low or medium
   Nuts—All high
   Misc.—Cereals—medium, except brown rice, wheat germ (high); and
   blackstrap molasses (high)
   Animals: All medium, except herring, salmon, liver (high)
   Microorganisms: All high or medium—yeast, intestinal bacteria (high);
   some other bacteria

2. **Dietary Sources**
   High: 1000-10,000 µg/100 g
   Liver (beef, calf, pork), herring, salmon
   Walnuts, peanuts, wheat germ, brown rice
   Yeast, blackstrap molasses
   Medium: 100-1000 µg/100 g
   Bananas, avocados, grapes, pears
   Barley, cabbage, carrots, corn, oats, peas, potatoes, rye, kale,
   tomatoes, turnips, yams, brussel sprouts, cauliflower, spinach,
   soybeans, wheat
   Beef, lamb, pork, veal (heart, brains, kidney); cod, flounder, halibut,
   mackerel, whale, sardines, tuna
   Butter, eggs
   Low: 10-100 µg/100 g
   Apples, cantaloupes, grapefruit, lemons, oranges, peaches, raisins,
   strawberries, watermelons, cherries, currants (red)
   Asparagus, beans, beet greens, lettuce, onions
   Cheese, milk

MEDICAL AND NUTRITIONAL ROLE

1. **Units:**   By weight, mg

2. **Normal Blood Levels:**   11.2 ug/100 ml

3. **Recommended Allowances**
   Children—0.5-1.2 mg/day*
   Adults—2.0 mg/day*
   Special—Pregnancy and lactation, 2.5 mg/day

* Depends on protein content of food and inborn errors of metabolism; irradiation increases need.

4. **Administration**
    Injection—Intravenous, subcutaneous
    Topical—No data
    Oral—Preferred route

5. **Factors Affecting Availability**
    Decrease
        Administration of isoniazid
        30-45% loss in cooking, water sol.
        Diuresis, G.I. diseases
        Irradiation
    Increase
        Intestinal bacterial production (very small amount)
        Storage in liver

6. **Deficiency Symptoms**
    General
        Cutaneous lesions
        Anemia
        Neuronal dysfunction including convulsions
        Increased excretion of xanthurenic acid
    Lab Animals
        Blood urea and urea excretion enhanced
        γ-globulin and hemoglobin decreased
        Urinary oxalate increased
        Insulin insufficiency
        Acrodynia
        Demyelinization of peripheral nerves
        Tonoclonic convulsion
        Adrenal—enlarged zona fasciculata
        Poor reproduction

7. **Effects of Overdose**
    Limited toxicity man (only at 3 g/kg dosage)
    Convulsions at 4 g/kg (rat)

METABOLIC ROLE

1. **Biosynthesis**
    Precursors—Possibly glycine, serine or glycolaldehyde
    Intermediates—Unknown

2. **Production:**   Species and Site
     Plants—Fungi, cereal germ, seeds
     Bacteria—Intestinal
     Animals—None

3. **Storage Site:**   Muscle phosphorylase (skeletal muscle) (small amount)

4. **Blood Carriers:**   Blood protein complexes

5. **Half-life:**   57% of ingested dose excreted per day

6. **Target Tissues:**   Nervous tissue, liver, lymph nodes, muscle tissue

7. **Reactions**
     Coenzyme forms—Codecarboxylase (pyridoxal-5-phosphate); pyridox-
         amine phosphate; Cu, Fe, Al chelates of coenzymes probably are
         active forms

Organ	Enzyme System	Effect
Liver	1. Transaminases (glutamic, aspartic)	Activated
Liver	2. Amino acid decarboxylases (histidine)	Activated
Liver	3. Tryptophan metabolism (kynureninase)	Activated
Liver	4. Tyrosine and phenylalanine metabolism	Activated
Muscle	5. Phosphorylases (constituent of)	Completed
Liver	6. Dehydrases (porphyrin synthesis, serine)	Activated
Liver	7. Racemases (alanine racemase)	Activated
Liver	8. Oxidases (diamine)	Activated
Liver	9. Desulfhydrases (cysteine)	Activated
Liver	10. Serine transhydroxymethylase	Activated

8. **Mode of Action**
     Cellular
         Anabolic—Unsaturated fatty acid biosynthesis
         Catabolic—Nonoxidative metabolic changes, decarboxylations, trans-
             aminations, glycogen phosphorylation
         Other—amino acid absorption and transport
     Organismal
         Growth, maintenance of adrenal cortex
         Production of niacin, norepinephrine, serotonin, histamine, acetyl-
             choline, γ-aminobutyric acid

Production of bile acids (taurine synthesis)

Erythrocyte formation, gluconeogenesis and glycogenolysis reactions

9. **Catabolism**

Intermediates—All converted to pyridoxal

Excretion products

Urine—4-pyridoxic acid (3-4 mg/day); pyridoxal (0.2-0.3 mg/day)

Feces—0.5-0.8 mg/day

MISCELLANEOUS

1. **Relationship to Other Vitamins**

Pantothenic acid—B_6 defic. results in lowered concentration of co-enzyme A

B_{12}—B_6 defic. results in reduced absorption and storage of B_{12}

Vitamin E—B_6 synergizes with E to control metabolism of unsaturated fats

Vitamin C—Excretion of C increased in B_6 deficiency, conversion of vit. C to oxalates increased, i.e., oxaluria. Helps alleviate some symptoms of B_6 deficiency. Synergizes with B_6 in tyrosine metabolism

Niacin—B_6 coenzyme for niacin synthesis from tryptophan, also synergistic

Vitamin B_1—Overdose of B_1 causes B_6 deficiency in rats, synergistic

Vitamin B_2—Synergistic in action with B_6

Biotin—Synergistic with B_6, B_2 and niacin in skin maintenance

2. **Relationship to Hormones**

Thyroxine—decreases the activity of various pyridoxalphosphate dependent enzyme systems

Insulin—Insufficiency of insulin in B_6 deficiency in animals

Norepinephrine, Acetylcholine, serotonin, epinephrine—B_6 involved in synthesis of these hormones

ACTH—Adrenal cortex zona fasciculata enlarged (hypertrophied) on B_6 deficiency

B_6 possibly involved in synthesis and function of these hormones (STH a synergist in growth)

STH

Estradiol-17β

Testosterone

FSH

LH

Cortisol
Aldosterone
Epinephrine
Glucagon

3. **Unusual Features**

Involved in dental caries, oxaluria

Linoleic acid relieves dermatitis symptoms of B$_6$ deficiency

Presence of B$_6$ in phosphorylase a and b in large amounts implicates glucagon, epinephrine, and norepinephrine in function of B$_6$

Great diversity of deficiency symptoms depending on species

Heavy metal ion involved in binding to enzyme

Involvement in stress, electrolyte balance, energy production, and water metabolism by unknown pathways

4. **Possible Relationships of Deficiency Symptoms to Metabolic Action**

Cutaneous lesions—Synergism of B$_6$ with niacin and B$_2$ for skin maintenance

Convulsions—Synergism of B$_6$ with B$_1$ involved in nervous tissue maintenance

Xanthurenic acid excretion—Kynureninase requires B$_6$ as coenzyme

Anemia—Synergism of B$_6$ with B$_{12}$ for anti-anemic action, maintenance of erythrocyte production

10
Vitamin B$_{12}$

GENERAL INFORMATION

1. **Synonyms:** Cobalamin, cyanocobalamin

2. **History**
   1926—Minot and Murphy controlled pernicious anemia using liver
   1944—Castle demonstrated intrinsic factor needed to control pernicious anemia with liver
   1948—Rickes *et al.* isolated and crystallized factor in liver controlling pernicious anemia
   1948—Smith and Parker crystallized and designated liver factor as vit. B$_{12}$
   1948—West demonstrated clinical activity of vit. B$_{12}$
   1955—Hodgkin *et al.* determined structure of vit. B$_{12}$

3. **Physiological Forms:** Hydroxocobalamin (vit. B$_{12a}$). Aquocobalamin (vit. B$_{12b}$)

4. **Active Analogs and Related Compounds**
   Nitrocobalamin (vit. B$_{12c}$), chlorocobalamin, thiocyanatocobalamin

5. **Inactive Analogs and Related Compounds (in Man)**
   ψ-Vitamin B, factors B, C, D, E, F, G, H, I

6. **Antagonists:** Methylamide, ethylamide, anilide, lactone derivatives, pteridine, nicotinamide

7. **Synergists:**   Vitamins A, E, C, B$_1$, folic acid, biotin, pantothenic acid,

8. **Physiological Functions**
   Coenzyme in nucleic acid, protein and lipid synthesis
   Maintain growth, nucleic acid synthesis, protein synthesis, lipid synthesis, and methylations
   Maintain epithelial cells and nervous system (myelin sheath), erythropoiesis (with folic acid) and leukopoiesis

9. **Deficiency Diseases, Disorders:**   Retarded growth, pernicious anemia, megaloblastic anemia, macrocytic, hyperchromic anemia, glossitis, spinal cord degeneration, sprue

10. **Sources for Species Requiring It**
    Required by most vertebrates, some protozoa, bacteria, algae
    Exogenous sources—Vertebrates, some bacteria, protozoa, algae (not available from intestinal bacteria in man)
    Endogenous sources—Bacteria, actinomycetes

CHEMISTRY

1. **Structure**

Vitamin B$_{12}$,
$C_{63}H_{90}CoN_{14}O_{14}P$

2. Reactions

Heat—Unstable   Oxidation—Unstable
Acid—Unstable   Reduction—Unstable
Alkali—Unstable   Light—Unstable
Water—Neutral

3. Properties

Appearance—red powder   Solubility
MW—1357 H_2O—1.25 g/100 ml
MP—Blackens at 190°C   Alc.—sol.
Crystal Form—Orthorhombic   Acet., Benz., Chl., Eth.—Insol.
  needles   Absn. Max.—278, 361,
Salts—Perchloric acid   550 mμ (H_2O)
Important Groups for activity $[\alpha]_D^{23} = -59°$ (aq. soln.)
  5,6-Dimethylbenzimidazole   Chemical Nature
  α-Ribothiazole   Polyacidic base
                                 Benzimidazole nucleotide
                                 Porphyrin-like corrin
                                 Reducing agent

4. Commercial Production

Fermentation of *S. griseus* or *S. aureofaciens*
By-product of antibiotic production

5. Isolation

Sources—Liver, fish solubles
Method
    Extract with aqueous alcohol
    Adsorb B_{12} on charcoal, elute with 65% alcohol
    Column chromatography on silica or alumina
    Wash with acetone, elute with alcohol
    Crystallize

6. Determination

Bioassay
    Microbial—*L. leichmanii, O. malhamensis, E. gracilis*
    Animal—Chick and rat—curative dose
Physicochemical—Spectrophotometry, polarography, isotope dilution

DISTRIBUTION AND SOURCES

1. **Occurrence**
   Plants: Vegetables—Very low—soybeans, green beans, beets, carrots, peas
   Nuts, seeds—Very low—oats, wheat
   Animals: All animals, especially in organs—Liver, kidney, heart, spleen,
   brain, stomach, intestine
   Eggs, milk
   Microorganisms: *S. aureofaciens, B. megatherium,* protozoa, soil
   bacteria, intestinal bacteria
   Miscellaneous: Sea water, sewage sludge

2. **Dietary Sources**
   High: 50 μg-500 μg/100 g
   Kidney (lamb, beef)
   Liver (lamb, beef, calf, pork)
   Brain (beef)
   Medium: 5-50 μg/100 g
   Kidney (rabbit)
   Liver (rabbit, chicken)
   Heart (beef, rabbit, chicken)
   Egg yolk
   Clams, sardines, salmon, crabs, oysters, herring
   Low: 0.5-5 μg/100 g
   Cod, flounder, haddock, halibut, lobster, scallop, shrimp, swordfish,
   tuna, whale
   Beef, pork lamb, chicken
   Cheeses, milk, eggs

MEDICAL AND NUTRITIONAL ROLE

1. **Units:**   1 USP = 1 μg vit. B$_{12}$ = 11,000 LLD units (*L. lactis Dorner* units)

2. **Normal Blood Levels (Man):**   0.08 μg/100 ml (0.03 μg/100 ml, serum)

3. **Recommended Allowances**
   Children—2-5 μg/day
   Adults—5-6 μg/day
   Special—Pregnancy, 8 μg/day; lactation, 6 μg/day; intestinal malabsorp-
   tion or disease; anorexia; old age; neuropathies; malnutrition;
   alcoholism

4. **Administration**

        Injection—Parenteral, intramuscular

        Topical—No data

        Oral—Not very effective unless intrinsic factor (enzyme) present

5. **Factors Affecting Availability**

        Decrease

            Cooking losses—Heat labile

            Cobalt deficiency (ruminants)

            Intestinal malabsorption or parasites

            Lack of intrinsic factor

            Intestinal disease, aging

            Vegetarian diet

            Excretion in feces

            Gastrectomy

        Increase

            Administration of sorbitol

            Synthesis by intestinal bacteria (not normally)

            Reduced temperature

            Food in stomach

6. **Deficiency Symptoms**

        Poor growth

        Increased hemolysis of RBC's

        Megaloblastic marrow

        Macrocytic, hyperchromic anemia

        Glossitis

        Degenerative changes in spinal cord, nervous symptoms

        Decreased blood and tissue lipids

        Disturbed carbohydrate metabolism—excretion of methylmalonic acid

        Leukopenia

        Gastrointestinal tract changes

        Loss of hatchability ⎫

        Poor feathering   ⎬ Chickens

        Reproductive failure ⎫

        Porphyrin whiskers ⎬ Rats

        Dermatitis   ⎫

        Impaired reproduction ⎬ Pigs

7. **Effects of Overdose, Excess**

        Polycythemia reported

        General lack of toxicity

METABOLIC ROLE

1. **Biosynthesis**
   Precursors
     Glycine—corrin nucleus
     δ-Aminolevulinic acid—corrin nucleus
     Methionine—corrin nucleus
   Intermediates
     Porphobilinogen
     α-d-Ribosides of benzimidazole
     5,6-Dimethylbenzimidazole
     α-Ribazole

2. **Production:**   Species—Bacteria (some); actinomycetes (some)

3. **Storage:**   Liver (30-60%), lungs, kidneys, spleen

4. **Blood Carriers:** α_1-Globulins (52%), α_2-globulins (21%), Albumins (16%), β-globulins (7%), γ-globulins (6%)

5. **Half-life:** > 1 year

6. **Target Tissues:**   Central nervous system, kidneys, myocardium, muscle, skin, bone

7. **Reactions**
   Coenzyme forms
     Adenyl cobamide coenzyme (adenyl nucleoside)
     5,6-Dimethylbenzimidazolylcobamide coenzyme
     Benzimidazolylcobamide coenzyme

Organ	Enzyme System	Effect
	MUTASES	
Liver	Glutamate mutase (glut—aspartic)	Activated
Liver	Methylmalonyl CoA mutase (methyl malonic—succinic)	Activated
	DEHYDRASES	
Liver	Diol dehydrase (glycerol-1,3-propanediol)	Activated
Liver	Glycerol dehydrase (glycerol-β-OH-propionaldehyde)	Activated
Liver	Ethanolamine deaminase (ethanolamine-ammonia, acetaldehyde)	Activated

	TRANSMETHYLASES	
Liver	$B_{1\,2}$ enzyme (homocysteine—methionine) with folate	Activated
Liver	Thymidine synthesis enzymes (purine biosynthesis)	Activated
	REDUCTASES	
Liver	Methane formation enzymes	Activated
Liver	Ribonucleotide reductase (ribonucleotide— deoxyribonucleotide)	Activated
Liver	Lysine fermentation enzymes	Activated
Liver	Acetate synthesis enzymes	Activated

8. **Mode of Action**
   Cellular
      Anabolic
         DNA synthesis (nucleolar methylations, ribotide conversion)
         RNA synthesis (purine synthesis, nucleolar methylation)
         Protein synthesis (DNA synthesis, methionine synthesis)
         Synthesis of lipids
         Porphyrin synthesis
         Anabolic action—mitosis and growth
         Choline synthesis
      Catabolic
         Carbohydrate metabolism (propionic acid)
         Lipid metabolism (glycerol, ethanolamine)
      Other
         Maintenance of membranes, esp. myelin sheath
         Maintenance of —SH groups in reduced form
   Organismal
      Maintains epithelial and mucosal cells
      Maintains normal bone marrow
      Maintains normal G.I. tract
      Maintains normal CNS
      Maintains erythropoiesis and leukopoiesis
      Maintains body lipids, lipotropic
      Maintains normal growth
      Improves nitrogen retention

9. **Catabolism**
   Intermediates—No body destruction
   Excretion products
      Urine—0.131 μg/day (free)

Feces—34% of ingested dose
Bile—Some reabsorption (enterohepatic recirculation)

MISCELLANEOUS

1. **Relationship to Other Vitamins**
   Folic acid—Active with B$_{12}$ in nucleic acid and methionine synthesis; combined action with vit. B$_{12}$; deficiency of F.A. increases B$_{12}$ absn.
   Vitamin A—Uptake and utilization of carotenes increased with B$_{12}$ in diet; maintenance of mucosal and epithelial cells
   Vitamin B$_6$—Deficiency reduces B$_{12}$ absorption in gut
   Biotin—Active with B$_{12}$ in methylmalonyl CoA metabolism
   Niacin—B$_{12}$ deficiency causes decrease in liver NAD
   Pantothenic acid—B$_{12}$ participates in methylmalonyl CoA conversion; has sparing action of B$_{12}$ and vice versa
   Riboflavin—Possible synthesis from 5,6-dimethylbenzimidazole moiety of B$_{12}$
   Vitamins E, C—Can substitute for vit. B$_{12}$ in certain conditions and synergize it; synergize vit. B$_{12}$ in treatment of macrocytic anemia
   Vitamin B$_1$—Synergistic to B$_{12}$

2. **Relationship to Hormones**
   T4-Deficiency of T4 impairs B$_{12}$ absorption
      Antithyroid antibodies in serum of B$_{12}$ deficient patients
      Increased T4 produces loss of B$_{12}$
   Parathormone—Pernicious anemia found coexisting with hypoparathyroidism (Ca metabolism)
   STH—B$_{12}$ needed for mitosis and growth (with folic acid)

3. **Unusual Features**
   Cyanide group an artifact of preparation
   The only vitamin synthesized in sizable amounts only by microorganisms (possibly in tumors)
   Only vitamin with metal ion
   Works with glutathione
   Glutathione content decreased on B$_{12}$ deficiency
   Mitosis retarded in B$_{12}$ deficiency
   Requires intrinsic factor (enzyme) for oral activity
   Increases tumor size (Rous sarcoma)
   Diamagnetic properties
   No acidic or basic groups revealed on titration (no pKa).

4. **Possible Relationships of Deficiency Symptoms to Metabolic Action**

Degenerative changes in spinal cord—decreased RNA synthesis

Megaloblastic marrow—decreased DNA synthesis (with folate)

Glossitis—decreased cell division of tongue cells

Macrocytic hyperchromic anemia—decreased DNA synthesis of precursor cells

Decreased blood and tissue lipids—possibly due to presence of plasma hemolytic factor in B_{12} deficiency

Disturbed CHO metabolism—activation of methylmalonic acid mutase by B_{12}

Leukopenia—decreased DNA synthesis in stem cells

GI tract changes—decreased cell division of gastric mucosal cells

Increased hemolysis—presence of plasma hemolytic factor in B_{12} deficiency

11
Ascorbic Acid

GENERAL INFORMATION

1. **Synonyms:** Vitamin C, antiscorbutic vitamin, cevitamic acid, hexuronic acid

2. **History**
   1757—Lind described scurvy
   1907—Holst and Frolich produced experimental scurvy
   1928—Zilva described antiscorbutic agents in lemon juice
   1928—Szent-Györgyi isolated hexuronic acid from lemon juice
   1932—Waugh and King identified hexuronic acid as antiscorbutic agent
   1933—Haworth established configuration of hexuronic acid
   1933—Reichstein synthesized hexuronic acid
   1933—Haworth and Szent-Györgyi changed name of hexuronic acid to ascorbic acid

3. **Physiological Forms:** l-Ascorbic acid, dehydroascorbic acid

4. **Active Analogs and Related Compounds:** l-Glucoascorbic acid, d-arabo-ascorbic acid, l-rhamnoascorbic acid, 6-desoxy-l-ascorbic acid

5. **Inactive Analogs and Related Compounds:** d-Ascorbic acid

6. **Antagonists:** d-Glucoascorbic acid, deoxycorticosterone

7. **Synergists:**   Vitamins A, E, B_{12}, B_6, K, pantothenic acid, testosterone, STH, folic acid

8. **Physiological Functions**
   Absorption of iron
   Cold tolerance, maintenance of adrenal cortex
   Antioxidant
   Metabolism of tryptophan, phenylalanine, tyrosine
   Growth
   Wound healing
   Synthesis of polysaccharides and collagen
   Formation of cartilage, dentine, bone, teeth
   Maintenance of capillaries

9. **Deficiency Diseases and Disorders:**   Scurvy, megaloblastic anemia of infancy

10. **Sources for Species Requiring It:**
    Most species require it (most make it)
    Exogenous sources—Primates, Guinea pig, Indian fruit bat, red vented bulbul, trypanosomes, yeast
    Endogenous sources—Remainder of vertebrates, invertebrates, plants, and some molds and bacteria

CHEMISTRY

1. **Structure**

Ascorbic Acid, $C_6H_8O_6$

2. **Reactions**
   Heat—Labile   Oxidation—Labile
   Acid—Stable   Reduction—Stable (reducing agent)
   Alkali—Labile   Light—Labile
   Water—Acid (pH 3) labile

3. **Properties**
   Appearance—White powder

MW—176.12

MP—190-192°C (decomp.)

Crystal Form—plates, needles

Salts—Ca, Na, metals

Important Groups for activity

    Lactone ring

    Enolic hydroxyls

Solubility

  H_2O—0.3 g/ml

  Acet., Alc.—Slightly sol.

  Benz., Chl., Eth.—Insol.

  Absn. Max.—245 mμ (acid)

            265 mμ (neutral)

  Redox Potential—E_0^1 = +0.166 volt

  (pH 4)

  Chemical Nature—Hexose acid

  α_D^{25} = +20.5° H_2O)

  Misc.—pKa_1 = 4.17

         pKa_2 = 11.57

4. Commercial Production

Microbiological—*Acetobacter suboxidans* oxidative fermentation of calcium d-gluconate.

Chemical—Oxidation of l-sorbose

5. Isolation

Sources—Adrenal cortex, citrus juices

Method—Ppt, from citrus juice as Pb-complex; crystallize from alcohol-petroleum ether

6. Determination

Bioassay—Guinea pig growth or tooth structure; serum alkaline phosphatase

Physicochemical—Titration against standard oxidizing dye solution, colorimetry of excess dye.

DISTRIBUTION AND SOURCES

1. Occurrence

Plants (High):

  Fruit—Strawberry, citrus, pineapple, guava, black currant, West Indian cherry

  Vegetables—Cabbage, turnip greens, tomatoes, broccoli, kale, horseradish, parsley, corn

  Nuts—English walnuts (green)

  Miscellaneous—Rose hips, molds

Animals: All-Retina > pituitary > corpus luteum > adrenal cortex > thymus > liver > brain > testes > ovaries > spleen > thyroid >

pancreas > saliv. glands > lungs > kidney > intestine > heart muscle > WBC > RBC > plasma

Microorganisms

No intestinal synthesis except in rat

Produced by certain molds

Required by bacteria, yeasts, and molds for multiplication

2. **Dietary Sources**

High: 100-300 Mg/100 g

Broccoli, brussel sprouts, collards, horseradish, kale, parsley, peppers (sweet), turnip greens

Black currant, guava, rose hips

Medium: 50-100 mg/100 g

Beet greens, cabbages, cauliflower, chives, kohlrabi, mustard, watercress, spinach

Lemons, oranges, papayas, strawberries

Low: 25-50 mg/100 g

Asparagus, lima beans, beet greens, chard, cowpeas, mint, okra, spring onions, peas, potatoes, radishes, rutabagas, turnips, dandelion greens, fennel, soybeans, summer squash

Gooseberries, passion fruit, grapefruit, limes, loganberries, mangoes, cantaloupes, honeydews, red currants, white currants, tangerines, raspberries, tomatoes, kumquats

MEDICAL AND NUTRITIONAL ROLE

1. **Units:**   1 I.U. = 1 U.S.P. unit = 0.05 mg l-ascorbic acid

2. **Normal Blood Levels:**   0.5-1 mg% (plasma), 25 mg% (white blood cells); vary with diet

3. **Recommended Allowances**

Children—40 mg/day

Adults—60 mg/day (males), 55 mg/day (females)

Special—Pregnancy (60 mg/day), lactation (60 mg/day); increased with infection, stress, trauma, allergies, old age, increased protein consumption

4. **Administration**

Injection—Intramuscular, intravenous

Topical—No data

Oral—Preferred route

5. **Factors Affecting Availability**
    Decrease
        Damage to adrenal cortex, presence of antagonists
        Food preparation (oxidation, storage, leaching, cooking)
    Increase
        Storage in body (adrenal cortex)
        Antioxidants, synergists in diet

6. **Deficiency Symptoms**
    General
        Hyperkeratotic papules on buttocks and calves
        Perifollicular hemorrhage, edema
        Wound healing failure
        Teeth and gum defects
        Weakness, listlessness, rough skin, aching joints
        Scorbutic bone formation
    Lab animals
        Anemia, loss of weight
        Abnormal collagen, no intercellular cement

7. **Effects of Overdose**
    None noted—Essentially nontoxic in man, except as noted below
    Possible kidney stones, in gouty individuals
    Inhibitory in excess doses on cellular level (mitosis inhibited)
    Possible damage to β-cells of pancreas and decreased insulin production
        by dehydroascorbic acid

METABOLIC ROLE

1. **Biosynthesis**
    Precursors—d-Mannose, d-fructose, glycerol, sucrose, d-glucose, or d-
        galactose
    Intermediates—UDP glucose, d-glucuronic acid, gulonic acid, l-gulono-
        lactone, (Mn^{++} cofactor)

2. **Production**—Species and Sites
    All animals (except primates, guinea pig, fruit bat, bulbul)—kidney and
        liver (rat—intest. bacteria supply)
    Plants (green leaves, fruit skin)
    Cell sites—Microsomes, mitochondria, golgi

3. **Storage Sites:**   Adrenal cortex (small amount)

4. **Blood Carriers:**   Free in blood, especially in white blood cells

5. **Half-life:**   16 days (man), few days (guinea pig)

6. **Target Tissues:**   Adrenal cortex, pituitary, ovary, connective tissue, bone, liver, teeth, gums

7. **Reactions**
   Coenzyme form: Redox couple—l-ascorbic $\rightleftharpoons$ dehydroascorbic acid

Organ	Enzyme Systems	Effect
	HYDROXYLATING	
Connective tissue	Proline → hydroxyproline (collagen synth.)	Activated
Liver	Tryptophan → 5-hydroxytryptophan (tryptophan metab.)	Activated
Adrenal cortex	Deoxycorticosterone → hydroxy-corticosteroids (steroid hormone synth.)	Activated
	OXIDATION-REDUCTION	
Liver	DPNH—cytochrome b_5 (electron transport)	Activated
Liver	Tyrosine—homogentisic acid (tyrosine metabolism)	Activated
Liver	Glutathione (reduction reaction)	Activated
Liver	Ascorbic acid oxidase (oxidation reactions)	Activated
Liver	Plasma iron—ferritin (reduction)	Activated
Liver	Amidases, proteases, glycosidases, peroxidases, esterases	Activated
Liver	Arginase, papain, liver esterase, catalase, cathepsin	Activated
Liver	Urease, b-amylase	Inhibited

8. **Mode of Action**
   Cellular
      Anabolic
         Collagen synthesis—Proline hydroxylation
         Steroid synthesis—Accelerates acetate incorp. into cholest.
         Serotonin, melanin synthesis
         Polysaccharide synthesis—Chondroitin sulfate incorp.
      Catabolic—Antimitotic agent

Other
    Cellular antioxidant—Maintains membranes
    Respiration—Cellular reductions and oxidations
    Maintenance of electron transport chain in mitochondria
    Maintains low redox level for vit. E and sulfhydryl enzymes
    Maintenance of peroxidase system (detoxification)
    Stimulates phagocytosis
Organismal
    Absorption of iron, ferritin production.
    Maintenance of adrenals and ovaries (hormone biosynthesis)
    Maintenance of connective tissues
    Maintenance of steroid endocrine glands
    Maintains stress and wound healing reactions
    Maintenance of cartilage, bone, and teeth
    Maintenance of capillaries, control hemorrhage
    Respiration—maintains oxygen turnover

9. **Catabolism**
    Intermediates—Diketogulonic acid, oxalic acid
    Excretion products
        Urine—12-14% excreted as l-ascorbic acid
               12-18% excreted as diketogulonic acid
               24-63% excreted as oxalic acid
        Also in feces, sweat, respiratory CO_2.

MISCELLANEOUS

1. **Relationship to Other Vitamins**
    Vitamin A—Depletion causes drop in plasma vit. C levels; protected by
        vit. C against oxidation
    Vitamin B_{12}—Replaced by vit. C in lactic acid bacteria; can be replaced
        or potentiated by vit. C
    Folic acid—Vitamin C decreases symptoms of folic acid deficiency;
        formation promoted by vit. C, stimulates formation of citrovorum
        factor (folinic acid)
    Pyridoxine—Pyridoxine-PO_4 and vit. C related to tyrosine metabolism
    Vitamin E—Decreased synthesis and excretion of vit. C in vit. E deficient
        animals; protected by vit. C agrainst oxidation
    Pantothenic acid—Compensated partly by vit. C in deficiency of
        pantothenic acid

2. **Relationship to Hormones**

   Serotonin—Produced from tryptophan under influence of vit. C

   Thyroxine—Cold survival capacity due to vit. C (mediated via thyroxine)

   Epinephrine, Norepinephrine—Produced from tyrosine under influence of vit. C; vit. C protects against oxidation

   Deoxycorticosterone—Depresses action of vit. C on growth of skeletal tissues

   Aldosterone, estradiol-17β, testosterone, cortisol—Vit. C stimulates conversion of deoxycorticosterone in adrenal cortex (maybe needed for steroid synthesis)

   Cortisone—Alleviates scorbutic symptoms in joints

   STH, ACTH, FSH, LH—High concentrations of vit. C noted in pituitary tissues; STH a synergist in growth

3. **Unusual Features**

   Only d-form active

   Antistress factor and anti-infection factor

   Activates terminal oxidases in respiratory systems

   Sensitivity to oxidation by heavy metals (e.g., Cu) hemochromogens, and quinones

   Ease of reversible oxidation

   Increased excretion due to barbiturates and drugs

   Increased synthesis of vit. C due to chloretone in vit. C deficient animals

   Production of H_2O_2 on aerobic oxidation

   Increases nitrogen assimilation by plants

   Protects tissues against ionizing radiation

4. **Possible Relationships of Deficiency Symptoms to Metabolic Action**

   Failure to produce intercellular cement—Decrease of mucopolysaccharide synthesis from glucuronic acid

   Hemorrhage—Weak intercellular fibers causing capillary fragility

   Poor tooth and gum structure—Decreased collagen, mucopolysaccharide synthesis; bacterial invasion

   Lethargy—Decreased supply of adrenocortical and adrenal hormones

   Edema—Decreased aldosterone synthesis and capillary fragility

   Weight loss—Possibly decreased growth hormone level

12
Biotin

GENERAL INFORMATION

1. Synonyms: Bios IIB, protective factor X, vit. H, egg white injury factor, CoR

2. History

1924—Miller fractionated yeast growth factor Bios into Bios, I, IIB, IIc

1933—Allison *et al.* isolated CoR (respiratory factor legume nodule bacteria)

1934—Lease and Parsons described egg white injury in chicks

1936—Kögl, Tonnis isolated growth stimulant from yeast, and egg yolk, and named it biotin

1940—György identified vit. H, CoR, and biotin as equivalent

1941—Williams *et al.* found egg white injury due to antivitamin, avidin (inactivates biotin)

1942—Du Vigneaud characterized and determined structure of biotin

1943—Harris synthesized biotin

3. Physiological Forms

d (or +) Biotin (*cis*-form) (β-isomer, *d*(β-biotin)*cis*)

Of 8 possible stereoisomers (4 *cis*, 4 *trans*), only one active: *d*-biotin (*cis*)

α and β-isomers based on orientation of isomeric side chains of *cis* and *trans* forms

4. **Active Analogs and Related Compounds**
    Desthiobiotin in some species
    dl-Oxybiotin (microorganisms, rats, chicks)
    Biotinol (in rats)
    Biotin sulfoxide (in some)
    Biocytin (in some)

5. **Inactive Analogs and Related Compounds**
    dl-Epibiotin (*cis*)
    dl-Allobiotin (*trans*)
    dl-Epiallobiotin (*trans*)
    l-Biotin (*cis*)
    α and β-Isomers of these

6. **Antagonists**
    Desthiobiotin in some forms
    Ureylene phenyl
    Homobiotin
    Ureylenecyclohexyl butyric and valeric acids
    Norbiotin
    Avidin
    Lysolecithin
    Biotin sulfone

7. **Synergists:**   Vitamins B_2, B_6, B_{12}, folic acid, pantothenic acid, STH,
        testosterone

8. **Physiological Functions**
    As coenzyme for
        Carboxylation reactions
        Pyruvic oxidase
        Decarboxylation of OAA, succinate, aspartate, malate
        Biosynthesis of aspartate, citrulline, unsaturated fatty acids
    Growth
    Maintenance of skin, hair, sebaceous glands, nerves, bone marrow, sex
        glands

9. **Deficiency Diseases and Disorders (Man)**
    Nonspecific dermatitis
    Seborrheic dermatitis in infants, furunculosis

10. **Sources for Species Requiring It**
     Most organisms require it
     Exogenous sources—Most vertebrates, invertebrates, some bacteria and
          fungi (intestinal bacteria supply needs of man)
     Endogenous sources—Higher plants, most fungi and bacteria

CHEMISTRY

1. **Structure**

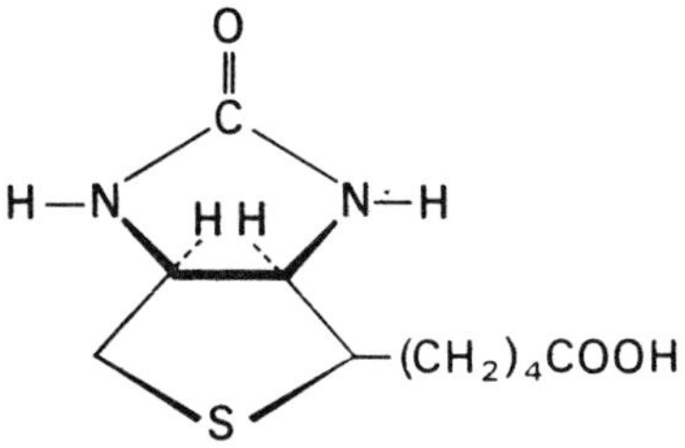

$d(\beta$-Biotin$)(cis)$, $C_{10}H_{16}N_2O_3S$

2. **Reactions**

Heat—Stable	Oxidation—Unstable
Acid—Unstable	Reduction—Forms desthiobiotin
Alkali—Unstable	Light—Stable
Water—Acidic	

3. **Properties**

Appearance—White powder
MW—244.3
MP—230-32°C
Crystal Form
    Orthorhombic (α)
    Colorless needles (β)
Salts—Na
Important Groups

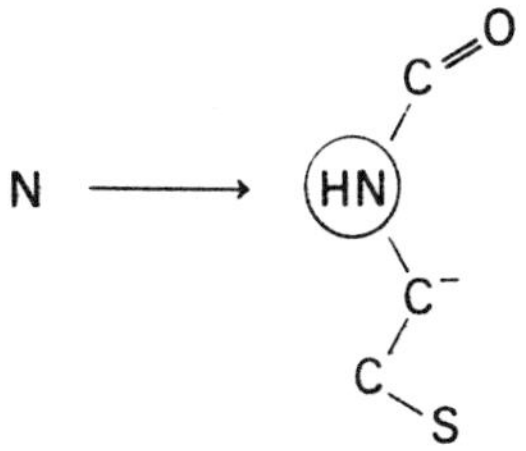

Solubility
    H_2O—0.03 g/100 ml
    Alc.—Sol.
    Acet., Benz. Chl. Eth.—Insol.
Absn. Max.—234 mμ
Chemical Nature
    Diamino-, monocarboxylic acid
    Substituted amino acid
Miscellaneous—pl = 3.5
    α_D^{21} = +91°   (0.1 N NaOH)

4. **Commercial Production**

   Use meso-diamino succinic acid derivative of fumaric acid for starting synthesis

5. **Isolation**

   Sources—Egg yolk, liver, milk

   Method—Extraction with acetone, precipitation with alc. and phospho-tungstate, adsorb and elute from charcoal, ppt. with $HgCl_2$, dissolve, purify, crystallize

6. **Determination**

   Bioassay

      Microbiological—*L. arabinosus*

      Rat and chick method—Growth response after biotin deficiency

   Physicochemical: Polarography

DISTRIBUTION AND SOURCES

1. **Occurrence**

   Plants

      Fruit—All low

      Vegetables—All low, except beans, peas, cauliflower

      Nuts—All medium, also cereals

   Animals: All low except in organs (esp. liver and kidneys are high)

   Microorganisms: Afford best source of biotin, especially yeast, lower fungi and bacteria

2. **Dietary Sources**

   High: 100-400 mg/100 g

      Royal jelly, yeast, lamb liver, pork liver

   Medium: 10-100 mg/100 g

      Wheat, rice, corn, oats, barley

      Eggs, beef liver, chicken, mushrooms

      Cowpeas, chick-peas, lentils, soybeans, cauliflower, chocolate

      Mackerel, salmon, sardines

      Almonds, peanuts, pecans, walnuts, filberts, hazelnuts

   Low: 0-1 mg/100 g

      Cheese, milk

      Apples, bananas, strawberries, cantaloupes, grapefruit, grapes, oranges, peaches, watermelon, avocados

Lima beans, beets, carrots, cabbages, corn, lettuce, onions, peas, sweet
potatoes, tomatoes, spinach, beet greens
Beef, lamb, veal, pork, tuna, halibut, oyster

MEDICAL AND NUTRITIONAL ROLE

1. **Units:** By weight, μg

2. **Normal Blood Levels:** 1.23 mg/100 ml (average)

3. **Recommended Allowances**
   Children—Unknown
   Adults—150-300 mg/day estimated. Sufficient supply from intestinal
     bacteria and diet

4. **Administration**
   Injection—parenteral, intramuscular
   Topical—No data
   Oral—Mainly used

5. **Factors Affecting Availability**
   Decrease
     Presence of avidin in food
     Cooking losses
     Antibiotics
     Sulfa drugs
     Binding in foods (yeast, animals)
   Increase: Synthesis by intestinal bacteria

6. **Deficiency Symptoms**
   General
     Desquamation of the skin
     Lassitude, somnolence, muscle pain
     Hyperesthesia
     Seborrheic dermatitis
   Alopecia, spastic gait, and kangaroo-like posture (rats and mice)
   Dermatitis and perosis (chicks and turkeys)
   Progressive paralysis, K^+ deficiency (dogs)
   Alopecia, spasticity of hind legs (pigs)
   Thinning and depigmentation of hair (monkeys)

7. **Effects of Overdose**
   None noted—1 g/kg not toxic
   Essentially nontoxic in man

METABOLIC ROLE

1. **Biosynthesis**
   Precursors—Pimelic acid, cysteine, carbamyl phosphate
   Intermediates—Desthiobiotin

2. **Production:**   Species and Sites
   Plants—Seedlings, leaves
   Fungi—Some
   Bacteria—Intestinal, some others

3. **Storage Sites:**   Liver

4. **Blood Carriers:**   Unknown

5. **Half-life:**   Requires 3-4 weeks to produce human deficiency with avidin

6. **Target Tissues:**   Skin, nervous tissue, male genitalia, bone marrow, liver, kidney

7. **Reactions**
   Coenzyme forms: CO_2-biotin-enz; d-biotin-lys-enz

Organ	Enzyme System	Effect
	CARBOXYLASES	
Liver	Propionyl-CoA carboxylase	Activated
	β-methylcrotonyl-CoA carboxylase	
	Acetyl-CoA carboxylase	
	Phosphoenolpyruvate carboxykinase	
	ATP-dependent pyruvic carboxylase	
	TRANSCARBOXYLASES	
Liver	Oxalosuccinate-acetyl-CoA transcarboxylase	Activated
	Methylmalonyl-oxalacetic transcarboxylase	
Liver	Malic enzyme	Activated
Liver	Ornithine transcarbamylase	Activated

8. **Mode of Action**

Cellular

Anabolic—Purine, protein, and carbohydrate synthesis; synthesis of aspartic acid, oleic acid, fatty acids

Catabolic—Deamination of serine in animals; tryptophan metabolism

Other—CO_2 fixation; ureido carbon of enzyme-bound biotin is the "active carbon"; implicated in carbamylation reactions

Organismal—Growth; maintenance of sebaceous glands, nervous tissue, skin, blood cells, hair, male genitalia

9. **Catabolism**

Intermediates—Little known

Excretion products

Urine—0.4 g/kg/day biotin, biocytin sulfoxide (?)

Feces—2.5 x amount in food intake (bacterial synthesis)

MISCELLANEOUS

1. **Relationship to Other Vitamins**

Pantothenic acid—Indicated by depigmentation of hair in deficiency of biotin + pantothenic acid

Vitamin C—ascorbic acid biosynthesis requires biotin

Vitamins B_2, B_6, niacin, A, D—Synergistic with biotin in maintenance of skin

Niacin—Not synthesized from tryptophan in biotin deficiency

Folic acid—(With pantothenic acid and biotin) increased stress response in adrenalectomized rats

2. **Relationship to Hormones**

Testosterone—Rat male genital system retarded in biotin deficiency (symptoms develop earlier than in female)

Cortisol—Adrenocortical insufficiency noted in biotin deficient rats.

STH—Synergist in growth

3. **Unusual Features**

Binding and inactivation by avidin protein found in egg white

Fetal tissues and cancer tissues are higher in biotin than adult tissues

Biotin deficiency increases severity and duration of some diseases notably some protozoan infections

Oleic acid and related compounds act to replace biotin as unspecific stimulatory compounds in bacteria

Combines to lysine residues of proteins
Only (+) isomer active
Inactivated by rancid fats, choline

4. **Possible Relationships of Deficiency Symptoms to Metabolic Action**

Desquamation of skin—Decreased fatty acid synthesis, synergism with A, D, other B vitamins

Hyperesthesia—Increased lactic acid levels

Lassitude, somnolence—Decreased oxidation of pyruvate

Muscle pain—Increased lactic acid levels, decreased fatty acid synthesis

Seborrheic dermatitis—Decreased synergism with vits. A, D, other B vitamins

13
Folic Acid

GENERAL INFORMATION

1. **Synonyms:** Folacin, pteroylmonoglutamic acid, antianemia factor, *L. casei* factor, vit. B_c, vit. M, PGA

2. **History**
   - 1931—Wills demonstrated a factor from yeast active in treating anemia
   - 1938—Day *et al.* found yeast or liver extracts active in treating anemia in monkeys
   - 1939—Hogan and Parrott prevented anemia in chicks with liver extract
   - 1940—Snell and Peterson isolated *L. casei* growth factor from liver and yeast
   - 1941—Hutchings *et. al.* found *L. casei* factor also essential for chicks
   - 1941—Mitchell, Snell, Williams isolated bacterial (*S. lactis R*) growth factor similar to *L casei* factor from yeast; named it folic acid
   - 1943—Stokstad reported *L. casei* factor from liver more active than that from yeast; evidence for multiple factors
   - 1946—Angier *et al.* isolated pteroylmonoglutamic acid, proved structure and synthesized it

3. **Physiological Forms:** Tetrahydrofolic acid, pteroyltriglutamic acid, pteroylheptaglutamic acid, l-folinic acid (citrovorum factor), dihydrofolic acid (5-formyl-5,6,7,8-tetrahydro-PGA) (leucovorin)

4. **Active Analogs and Related Compounds:** Pteroic acid (bacteria), 10-formyl-FAH_4, 5,10-methenyl-FAH_4, diopterin, 5,10-methylene-FAH_4, 5-formimino-FAH_4, rhizopterin (bact.), xanthopterin (bact.), biopterin (urine), ichthyopterin (fish), leucopterin (invertebrates)

5. **Inactive Analogs and Related Compounds:** d-folinic acid

6. **Antagonists:** Aminopterin (4-amino-PGA), methotrexate (amethopterin) pyrimethamine, 4-amino-pteroylaspartic acid

7. **Synergists:** Biotin, pantothenic acid, niacin, Vits. B_6, B_2 C, B_1, E, B_{12}, STH, estradiol, testosterone

8. **Physiological Functions:** Synthesis of nucleic acid, coenzyme in purine-pyrimidine metabolism, serine-glycine conversion, intermediate in metabolism of purines and pyrimidines, differentiation of embryonic nervous system, one-carbon transfer mechanisms, metabolism of tyrosine and histidine, formation of active formate, and methionine, synthesis of choline

9. **Deficiency Diseases and Disorders:** Anemias (macrocytic, megaloblastic, pernicious), glossitis, diarrhea, G.I. lesions, intestinal malabsorption, sprue

10. **Sources for Species Requiring It**
     Most animals require it
     Exogenous sources—Vertebrates, invertebrates, some bacteria (intestinal bacteria provide it in man, rats, dogs, pigs, rabbits) required by monkey, guinea pig, mice, fox, chicken, geese, turkeys
     Endogenous sources—Intestinal bacteria, fungi, yeast

CHEMISTRY

1. Structure

Pteridine   p-amino-   Glutamic
                     benzoic   acid
                     acid

Folic acid, $C_{19}H_{19}N_7O_6$

2. Reactions

Heat—Labile (in soln.)   Oxidation—Labile
Acid—Labile   Reduction—Stable
Alkali—Stable   Light—Labile (in soln.) to UV
Water—Stable (acid, pH 4.4)

3. Properties

Appearance—yellow crystals   Solubility
MW—441.2 H_2O—0.01 mg/ml
MP—Chars at 250°C   Acet., Alc.—Insol.
Crystal Form—Lenticular   Benz., Chl., Eth.—Insol.
Salts—Ba, Na, Pb   Absn. Max.—282, 350 mμ
Important Groups for activity   (pH 7.0)
  Glutamic acid   Misc.—pK_a = 8.2
  N^{10}, N^5, N^3, N^8 $\alpha_D{}^{25}$ = ±23° (0.1 N NaOH)
                                   Chemical Nature—Purine, amino
                                     acid, benzoic acid

4. Commercial Production

Extraction from yeast or liver; synthetic

5. Isolation

Sources—Spinach, liver, yeast, alfalfa, wheat bran
Method
  Extract (aq.) liver at pH 3.0
  Adsorb on norite, elute with NH_4OH-ethanol

Adsorb on superfiltrol pH 1.3, elute with NH_4OH-ethanol
Ppt. with Ba^{++}, pH 7.0 in alcohol
Esterify with methanol, extract with n-butanol
Adsorb on superfiltrol pH 7, elute ester with 75% acetone
Crystallize from hot methanol, hydrolyze ester
Recrystallize from hot H_2O

6. **Determination**
   Bioassay
   Animal—chick feathering, rat oviduct development
   Microbial—Growth of *L. casei, S. fecalis*
   Physicochemical
   Enzymatic—DPNH reductase activity
   Fluorometric—Fluorescence at 470 mμ
   Colorimetric—Estimate aromatic amine on cleavage
   Polarographic—Paper chromatography

DISTRIBUTION AND SOURCES

1. **Occurrence**
   Plants: Fruit—Low
   Vegetables—Green leafy vegetables, dried beans
   Nuts—Almonds, filberts, peanuts, walnuts
   Miscellaneous—Green leaves, grass, barley, oats, rye, wheat
   Animals
   Liver, kidney
   Butterflies (wing pigment, xanthopterin)
   Fish scales (ichthyopterin)
   Microorganisms: Intestinal bacteria, yeast, fungi, algae
   Miscellaneous: Mushrooms

2. **Dietary Sources**
   High: 90-300 mg/g
   Liver (beef, lamb, pork, chicken)
   Asparagus, spinach
   Wheat, bran
   Dry beans (lentils, limas, navy)
   Yeast
   Medium: 30—90 mg/100 g
   Kidney (beef)

Lima beans, snap beans, broccoli, corn, beet greens, chicory, endive, kale, parsley, chard, turnip greens, watercress

Almonds, filberts, peanuts, walnuts

Barley, oats, rye, wheat

Low: 0-30 mg/100 g

Beef (muscle, heart), lamb, pork, chicken, turkey (muscle)

All fruit tested

Cheese, milk

Brazil nuts, coconuts, pecans

Wax beans, beets, brussel sprouts, cabbages, carrots, brown rice, cauliflower, celery, cucumbers, eggplant, escarole, mustard, kohlrabi, lettuce, mushrooms, okra, onions, parsnips, peas, peppers, potatoes, pumpkins, radishes, rutabagas, squash, sweet potatoes, tomatoes, turnips

MEDICAL AND NUTRITIONAL ROLE

1. **Units:**   By weight, mg

2. **Normal Blood Levels:**   3.53 μg/100 ml (humans)

3. **Recommended Allowances**
   Children and adults
   0.4 mg/day estimate
   Provided by intestinal synthesis in man
   Required by monkey, guinea pig, mice, fox, chicken, geese, turkeys
   Special—Pregnancy, illness

4. **Administration**
   Injection—subcutaneous
   Topical—No data
   Oral—Preferred route

5. **Factors Affecting Availability**
   Decrease
   High urinary excretion (75% ingested)
   Destruction by certain intestinal bacteria
   Increased urinary excretion caused by vit. C
   Sulfonamides block intestinal synthesis
   Poor absorption

Increase—Intestinal bacterial synthesis and release: man, rats, dogs, pigs, rabbits

6. **Deficiency Symptoms**
    Intestinal disturbances
    Leucopenia
    Glossitis
    Thrombocytopenia
    Macrocytic anemia
    Pernicious anemia
    Sprue
    Megaloblastic erythropoiesis
    Gingivitis, agranulosis (monkey)
    Hydrocephalus, splenic enlargement (rats)
    Endocrine disturbances, poor feathering (chick)
    Lethargy, convulsions (guinea pig)

7. **Effects of Overdose**
    Man—No toxicity reported
    Mice—Renal damage, convulsions: LD_{50} = 600 mg/kg
    Chick—Arrest cells in metaphase with high doses

METABOLIC ROLE

1. **Biosynthesis**
    Precursors: Paraminobenzoic acid, glutamic acid, unknown pteridine
    Intermediates: Paraminobenzoylglutamic acid

2. **Production:**   Species and Sites
    Plants—Leaves, seeds, cereal germ, algae
    Bacteria—Intestinal supply sufficient for man, rats, pigs, dogs, rabbits; Other species require exogenous sources
    Fungi—yeast

3. **Storage:**   Liver (small amount)

4. **Blood Carriers:**   Prefolic acid A

5. **Half-life:**   75% of ingested folic acid excreted in urine in 24 hr

6. **Target Tissues:**   Liver, bone marrow, lymph nodes, kidneys

7. Reactions

Coenzyme forms: Folinic acid (citrovorum factor), 10-formyl-FH_4, 5,10-methylene-FH_4,   5-formimino-FH_4,   10-formimino-FH_4, 5-methyl-FH_4, 5-hydroxymethyl-FH_4

Organ	Enzyme System	Effect
Liver	REDUCTASES Dihydrofolate reductase: $FH_2 \rightarrow FH_4$ $N^5 N^{10}$-Methylene-FH_4 reductase: $N^5 N^{10}$-methylene-$FH_4 \rightarrow N^5$-methyl-FH_4	Activated
Liver	TRANSFERASES Formiminoglutamate formimino transferase: Formation of formimino glutamate Serine transhydroxymethylase: Glycine-serine interconversion Formylglutamate formyl transferase: Formation of glutamate	Activated
Liver	ISOMERASES N^5-formyl-tetrahydrofolate isomerase: N^5-formyl-$FH_4 \rightarrow N^{10}$-formyl-FH_4	Activated
Liver	SYNTHETASES Formyl tetrahydrofolate synthetase: $FH_4 \rightarrow N^{10}$-formyl-FH_4	Activated
Liver	CONJUGASES Folic acid conjugase: Converts pteroyltriglutamate $\rightarrow$ PGA	Activated

8. Mode of Action

Cellular
    Anabolic
        Purine and pyrimidine synthesis
        Choline synthesis
        Methionine synthesis
        Formation of lignin, nicotine, betaine
    Catabolic—Histidine metabolism, tryptophan metabolism
    Other
        Mitotic step: Metaphase $\rightarrow$ anaphase requires folic acid
        Serine-glycine interconversion
        Formiminoglutamate formation
Organismal
    Erythropoiesis, growth
    Maintenance of sex organs
    Maintenance of intestinal tract

Leukopoiesis
Differentiation of nervous system

9. Catabolism

Intermediates: Xanthopterin, leucopterin

Excretion products: Urine—Biopterin, leucovorin, pteroylglutamic acid, 10.8 μg/day (humans); feces—enterohepatic circulation of folate

MISCELLANEOUS

1. Relationship to Other Vitamins

Vitamin C

Facilitates conversion of folic to folinic acid (CF-citrovorum factor)

Protects folinic acid from oxidation, increases urinary excretion of CF

Fundamental role with folic acid in erythropoiesis

Vitamin B_{12}

Blood and marrow changes in pernicious anemia respond to folic acid or B_{12}

Neurological changes in pernicious anemia involve B_{12} and folic acid

Involved with folic acid in formation of methionine from homocysteine

Biotin—Aids in storage and utilization of pantothenic acid in liver, (with folic acid)

Pantothenic acid—Utilization in CoA synthesis (with biotin and folic acid)

Niacin

Need folic acid for niacin metabolism

DPNH required for production of N^5-methyl-FH_4

DPN involved in methionine formation (with folic acid)

Vitamin B_6—Required with folic acid for serine-glycine transformations and for methionine formation

Riboflavin—Required with DPN, folic acid, vit. B_{12}, vit. B_6, for methionine formation

2. Relationship to Hormones

Estradiol—Folic acid deficiency eliminates normal response of female reproductive organs to estrogens; pregnancies not normal

Testosterone—Folic acid increases action of testosterone on development of accessory sex organs

STH—Synergist in growth

3. **Unusual Features**
   Folic acid antagonists used in cancer therapy with temporary remissions
   Occurs in chromosomes
   Distributed throughout cell
   Needed for mitotic step metaphase $\rightarrow$ anaphase
   Antibody formation decreased in folic acid deficiency
   Choline-sparing effects
   Analgesic in man—pain threshold increased
   Low intravenous toxicity in man
   Antisulfonamide effects
   Enterohepatic circulation of folate
   Synthesized by psittacosis virus
   Concentrated in spinal fluid

4. **Possible Relationships of Deficiency Symptoms to Metabolic Action**
   Cytopenia—Decreased nucleic acid synthesis and porphyrin synthesis
   Intestinal disturbances—Indirect relationship with other vitamin deficiencies
   Thrombocytopenia—Decreased nucleic acid synthesis
   Leukopenia—Decreased nucleic acid synthesis
   Glossitis—Indirect effect of other vit. B deficiencies
   Macrocytic anemia and pernicious anemia—Vitamin B_{12} lack and decreased porphyrin synthesis
   Sprue—Indirect effect of lack of other vitamins

14
Niacin

GENERAL INFORMATION

1. Synonyms: Nicotinic acid, nicotinamide, P-P factor, antipellagra factor, anti-blacktongue factor, B_4

2. History
1867—Huber first synthesized nicotinic acid
1914—Funk isolated nicotinic acid from rice polishings
1915—Goldberger demonstrated that pellagra is a nutritional deficiency
1917—Chittenden and Underhill demonstrated that canine blacktongue is similar to pellagra
1935—Warburg and Christian determined niacinamide essential in hydrogen transport as DPN
1936—Euler *et al.* isolated DPN and determined its structure
1937—Elvhehjem *et al.* cured blacktongue with niacinamide from liver
1937—Fouts *et al.* cured pellagra with niacinamide
1947—Handley and Bond established conversion of tryptophan to niacin by animal tissues

3. Physiological Forms: Niacinamide, NAD (DPN, CoI), NADP (TPN, CoII), N^1-methylnicotinamide

4. Active Analogs and Related Compounds: Niacin esters, coramine, β-picoline, 3-hydroxymethylpyridine

5. Inactive Analogs and Related Compounds: Trigonelline

6. **Antagonists:**   Pyridine-3-sulfonic   acid   (bacteria),   3-acetylpyridine,
6-aminonicotinamide, 5-thiazole carboxamide

7. **Synergists:**   Vitamins B_1, B_2, B_6, B_{12}, D, pantothenic and folic acids, STH

8. **Physiological Functions:**   Maintenance of NAD, NADP; hydrogen and
electron transfer agents in CHO metabolism; furnish coenzymes for
dehydrogenase systems; coenzyme in lipid catabolism, oxidative
deamination, photosynthesis

9. **Deficiency Diseases, Disorders:**   Pellagra (man), blacktongue (dogs), malnutrition, dermatosis (man)

10. **Sources for Species Requiring It**
Required by all species:
Exogenous sources: Animals, some bacteria and fungi (not available from
intestinal bacteria in man, but some conversion from tryptophan
occurs in tissues)
Endogenous sources: Plants: algae, some bacteria and fungi. Animals:
(some species partly via tryptophan; other species completely via
tryptophan)

CHEMISTRY

1. **Structure**

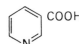
COOH   Niacin, $C_6H_5O_2N$

2. **Reactions**

Heat—Stable	Oxidation—Stable
Acid—Stable	Reduction—Unstable
Alkali—Stable	Light—Stable
Water—Acidic	

3. **Properties**

Appearance—White crystalline powder	Salts—HCl, metallic, Na
	Important Groups for activity
MW—123.1	—N on ring
MP—234-237°C (sublimes)	—COOH
Crystal Form—needles	

Solubility
 H_2O—1 g/100 ml
 Alc.—Sol.
 Benz., Chl., Eth., Acet.—Insol.
 Absn. Max.—261.5 mμ

Chemical Nature—Carboxylic
 acid; amine; substituted
 pyridine
Misc.—pKa = 4.8, 12.0
α_D = 0 (inactive)

4. **Commercial Production**
 Hydrolysis of 3-cyanopyridine
 Oxidation of nicotine, quinoline, or collidine

5. **Isolation**
 Sources—Liver, yeast
 Method—Remove lipids with solvents; hydrolyze with acid or alkali; extract niacin from acidified hydrolyzate; isolate as an acid, ester, or Cu salt; purify by recrystallization or sublimation

6. **Determination**
 Bioassay
 Animal—Dogs, blacktongue (curative)
 Microbial—*L. arabinosus*, growth
 Physicochemical
 Colorimetric—Cyanogen Br + reducing agent → color
 Spectrophotometric—UV max. of DPN, TPN

DISTRIBUTION AND SOURCES

1. **Occurrence**
 Plants:
 Fruit—All low (exc. avocados and dried figs, dates, and prunes—medium)
 Vegetables—All low (exc. beans, peas, potatoes, broccoli, asparagus, corn, parsley, kale—medium)
 Nuts—All medium (exc. coconuts, pecans—low)
 Animals: All medium [exc. livers, kidneys, beef heart, rabbit, turkey and chicken (white meat), tuna, halibut, swordfish—high]
 Microorganisms—All high—intestinal bacteria, some other bacteria

2. **Dietary Sources**
 High: 10,000-100,000 μg/100 g (10-100 mg/100 g)
 Peanuts (roasted), rice bran
 Liver (beef, calf, chicken, pork, sheep)

Heart (calf), kidney (pork, beef)

Rabbit, turkey and chicken (white meat)

Meat extract

Tuna, halibut, swordfish

Yeast

Medium: 1000-10,000 µg/100 g (1-10 mg/100 g)

Avocados, dates (dry), figs (dry), prunes (dry)

Asparagus, beans (kidney, lima, snap, wax), broccoli, corn, kale, lentils (dry), parsley, peas, potatoes, soybeans (dry)

Almonds (dry), cashew nuts, chestnuts, walnuts

Barley, oats, wheat, rye, brown rice, wheat germ, molasses, cheeses (camembert, swiss, roquefort)

Beef, veal, chicken (dark meat), duck, lamb, fish (exc. tuna, halibut, swordfish), clams, shrimp, oysters

Mushrooms

Low: 100-1000 µg/100 g (0.1-1.0 mg/100 g)

Apples, apricots, bananas, berries (black-, blue-, cran-, rasp-, straw-), cherries, currants, figs, grapes, grapefruit, lemons, melons, oranges, peaches, pears, pineapples, plums, raisins (dry), tangerines

Beets, beet greens, brussels sprouts, cabbage, carrots, cauliflower, celery, chicory, endive, cucumbers, dandelion greens, eggplant, kohlrabi, lettuce, onions, parsnips, peppers, pumpkins, radishes, rhubarb, spinach, sweet potatoes, tomatoes, turnips, watercress

Coconuts, pecans

Eggs, milk

MEDICAL AND NUTRITIONAL ROLE

1. **Units**—By weight, mg equivalents

2. **Normal Blood Levels:**   0.42-0.84 mg/100 ml

3. **Recommended Allowances**

Children—8-15 mg equivalents/day[*]

Adults—18 mg equivalents/day—male[*]; 13 mg equivalents/day—female[*]

Special—Pregnancy, 15 mg equivalents/day; lactation, 20 mg equivalents/day

---

[*] Depends on tryptophan content of diet; allow 10 mg equivalents for each 600 mg dietary tryptophan; assume 60 g/day protein in diet has 600 mg tryptophan.

4. **Administration**
   Injection—I.V.
   Topical—No data
   Oral—Preferred route

5. **Factors Affecting Availability**
   Decrease
   Cooking losses
   Bound form in corn, greens, seeds, partially unavailable
   Oral antibiotics
   Decreased absorption—disease
   Decreased tryptophan converted in B_6 deficiency
   Increase
   Alkali treatment of cereals
   Storage in liver, possibly muscle, kidney
   Increased intestinal synthesis

6. **Deficiency Symptoms**
   General (man)—Pellagra
   Retarded growth, achlorhydria
   Weakness, anorexia, indigestion, lassitude, dermatitis, pigmentation, diarrhea, tongue erythema, irritability, headaches, insomnia, memory loss
   Histological changes in CNS (dog, cat—blacktongue)
   Drooling (dog, cat—blacktongue)
   Perosis (chickens)
   Poor feathering (chickens)

7. **Effects of Overdose**
   Man—Limited toxicity starting approx. 1-4 g/kg dosage with individual variations in sensitivity. Burning, itching skin, peripheral vasodilation, decreased serum cholesterol, fatty liver, stimulated CNS, increased (pulse rate, respiratory rate, cerebral blood flow), decreased blood pressure
   Rat—Respiratory paralysis, ketosis
   Dogs—Death
   Chick—Inhibition of growth, fatty liver

METABOLIC ROLE

1. **Biosynthesis**
    Precursors—Tryptophan (animals, bacteria). Glycerol and succinic acid (plants)
    Intermediates—Kynurenine, hydroxyanthranilic acid, quinolinic acid

2. **Production:**   Species and Sites
    Fungi—*Neurospora*
    Plants—Leaves, germinating seeds, shoots
    Bacteria—Intestinal
    Animals—Tissues (not intestinal)

3. **Storage:**   Liver, heart, muscle

4. **Blood Carriers:**   Mostly as DPN in blood corpuscles

5. **Half-life**—1/3 of intake excreted in 24 hr

6. **Target Tissues:**   Liver (storage), heart, muscle, kidney, skin, G.I. tract, spinal cord

7. **Reactions**
    Coenzyme forms—(DPN,NAD) and (TPN,NADP). Act as redox couples: oxid $\leftrightharpoons$ reduced)

Organ	Enzyme System	Effect
	More than 50 metabolic reactions known	
Liver	DEHYDROGENASES: Alcohol, lactate, malate, isocitrate, glucose-6-P-succinic, β-hydroxy-butyrate, 3β-hydroxysteroids, betaine aldehyde, glutamate, α-glycerophosphate, uridine DPG, reduced glutathione, glyceraldehyde-3-P	Activated
Liver	OXIDASES: α-keto glutaric oxidase microsomal mixed function oxidases (DPN + TPN), oxidation of steroids, fatty acids, drugs and carcinogens	Activated or completed

8. **Mode of Action**
    Cellular
        Anabolic—Maintains microsomal reductive biosynthesis; photosynthesis

Catabolic
  Furnishes coenzymes for lipid catabolism
  Oxidative deamination
  CHO metabolism—Dehydrogenation, oxidation
  Key reactions in glycolysis, TCA cycle, and HMP
Other
  Hydrogen and electron transfer agent
  A mobile hydrogen transfer agent
  Maintains respiratory chain in mitochondria
Organismal
  Maintains growth
  Maintains energy supply to organism from degradation of carbo-
    hydrates, proteins, and lipids
  Maintains terminal section of respiratory cycle
  Maintains manufacture of hormones (steroids) proteins, lipids
  Stimulates gastric secretion and bile secretion

9. **Catabolism**
  Intermediates—N^1-Methylnicotinamide (liver)
  Excretion Products
    Feces: Nicotinic acid
    Urine: N^1-Methylnicotinamide; N^1-methyl-6-pyridone-3-carboxamide

MISCELLANEOUS

1. **Relationship to Other Vitamins**
  Vitamin B_2—Flavo-proteins reoxidize NAD, NADP
  Vitamin B_6—Decreased tryptophan conversion to niacin in B_6 deficiency
  Vitamins B_1, B_2, B_6, Pantothenic Acid, Folic Acid, Vitamin B_{12}—
    General synergism with niacin in alleviating deficiencies and in CHO
    metabolism
  Vitamins B_1, B_2, B_6—Needed for conversion of tryptophan to niacin

2. **Relationship to Hormones**
  Serotonin—Reduces tryptophan conversion to niacin (in cancer cases)
  Thyroxine, Insulin—Affect mitochondrial metabolism (as do DPN and
    TPN), and energy production from CHO metabolism
  Cortisol, Testosterone, Estradiol, Progesterone, Aldosterone—DPN and
    TPN involved in steroid oxidations in liver, in steroid hormone
    synthesis, and in cholesterol metabolism
  STH—Synergist in growth

3. **Unusual Features**

> Has hormonal quality, being partially internally synthesized
> Vasodilator, causes flushing (not as niacinamide)
> High corn diets cause deficiency due to tryptophan deficiency in corn protein and unavailability of niacin in corn
> Prepared from nicotine using strong oxidizing agent
> Stereospecific action of dehydrogenases on DPN
> Serum cholesterol lowering with large doses
> Antagonist (6-aminonicotinamide) active against some rat tumors
> Other pyridine derivatives functional in DPN and TPN
> Conversion of tryptophan not in intestines
> Toxicity of overdose preventable by feeding methionine (rats)

4. **Possible Relationships of Deficiency Symptoms to Metabolic Action**

> Retarded growth—General synergism of all B vitamins
> Dermatitis, itching, pigmentation, tongue lesions; other B vitamins, esp. B_2, involved
> Irritability, mental disturbances, nervous lesions related to thiamine synergism with niacin
> G.I. lesions and disturbances related to thiamine deficiency and synergism
> Mottled liver, fatty liver are disturbances of cholesterol metabolism

15
Pantothenic Acid

GENERAL INFORMATION

1. Synonyms: Chick antidermatitis factor, B3, Bios IIa, antigray-hair factor

2. History

1901—Wildiers described Bios, essential for yeast growth

1933—Williams isolated crystalline Bios from yeast; named it pantothenic acid

1938—Williams isolated pantothenic acid from liver

1939—Jukes determined liver antidermatitis factor (chick) identical to yeast factor

1939—Woolley *et al.* demonstrated β-alanine a vital part

1940—Harris, Folkers, *et al.* reported structure determination and synthesis of pantothenic acid; crystallization also

1950—Lipmann *et al.* discovered CoA

1951—Lynen characterized coenzyme A structure

3. Physiological Forms: Coenzyme A, pantotheine, d(+)pantothenic acid

4. Active Analogs and Related Compounds: Pantothenyl alcohol, β-alanine (bacteria), pantotheine (LBF), pantothine, pantothenylcystine, ethylmonoacetylpantothenate, ethyl pantothenate

5. Inactive Analogs and Related Compounds: l-pantothenate, α-alanine analogs

6. **Antagonists:** Pantoyltaurine, ω-methylpantothenic acid, bis(β-pantoyl-aminoethyl)disulfide, 6-mercaptopurine, pantoylaminoethanethiol

7. **Synergists:** Biotin, folic acid, vit. C, B_{12}, B_1, B_2, niacin, STH

8. **Physiological Functions:** Part of coenzyme A in carbohydrate metabolism (2 carbon transfer-acetate, or pyruvate), lipid metabolism (biosynthesis and catabolism of fatty acids, sterols, + phospholipids), protein metabolism (acetylations of amines & amino acids), porphyrin metabolism, acetylcholine production, isoprene production

9. **Deficiency Diseases, Disorders:** Dermatitis (chick), achromotrichia (rat), adrenal necrosis (rats), bloody whiskers (rat), alopecia (mice)

10. **Sources for Species Requiring It**
    All organisms require it
    Endogenous sources—Higher plants
    Exogenous sources—All other organisms (not available from intestinal synthesis in man)

CHEMISTRY

1. **Structure**

$$H-O-\overset{\overset{\displaystyle H}{|}}{\underset{\underset{\displaystyle H}{|}}{C}}-\overset{\overset{\displaystyle CH_3}{|}}{\underset{\underset{\displaystyle CH_3}{|}}{C}}-\overset{\overset{\displaystyle OH}{|}}{\underset{\underset{\displaystyle H}{|}}{C}}-\overset{\overset{\displaystyle O}{\|}}{C}-\overset{\overset{\displaystyle H}{|}}{N}-\overset{\overset{\displaystyle H}{|}}{\underset{\underset{\displaystyle H}{|}}{C}}-\overset{\overset{\displaystyle H}{|}}{\underset{\underset{\displaystyle H}{|}}{C}}-COOH$$

d(+)-Pantothenic acid, $C_9H_{17}O_5N$

Pantoic acid β-Alanine

2. **Reactions**

   Heat—Labile
   Acid—Labile (warm)
   Alkali—Labile (warm)
   Water—Sol. (acid)

   Oxidation—Stable
   Reduction—Stable
   Light—No data

3. **Properties**

   Appearance—yellow viscous oil
   MW—219.24

   MP—unstable
   Crystal Form—No data

Salts—Calcium, sodium
Important Groups for activity
   β-amino group
Solubility
   H_2O—7 g/100 ml
   Acet., Alc.—Sol.
   Benz., Chl., Eth.—Insol.

Absn. Max.—358 mμ
Chem. Nature—Conjugated amino
   acid, polyhydroxy acid
Miscellaneous:
   $\alpha_D{}^{25}$ = (+37.5°) (H_2O)
   pKa = 4.4

4. **Commercial Production:**   Synthetic
   Condensation of d-pantolactone with salt of β-alanine

5. **Isolation**
   Sources—Rice, bran, liver, yeast
   Method
      Extract liver with 90% ethyl alc.
      Adsorb out organic bases on Fuller's earth
      Adsorb vitamin on charcoal, pH 3.6, elute with ammonia
      Form brucine salts, extract selectively with $CHCl_3$
      Convert brucine salt to calcium salt
      Purify by fractional ppt. from organic solvents

6. **Determination**
   Bioassay
      Animal—Growth rate of chicks
      Microbiol—Growth of *L. casei*
   Physicochemical—Estimate of β-alanine after hydrolysis; estimate CoA
      by citrate cleavage enzyme

DISTRIBUTION AND SOURCES

1. **Occurrence**
   Plants
      Fruit—All (low)
      Vegetables—All (medium and low)
      Nuts—All (high and low)
   Animals
      All (medium and high)
      Organs (brain, heart, kidney, liver)
   Microorganisms
      Yeast (high), Rumen bacteria in sheep and cattle
      Molds

2. **Dietary Sources**
    High: 2.0 mg-10.0 mg/100 g
        Beef (brain, heart, liver, kidney), pork (liver, kidney), sheep liver, chicken liver, lamb kidney
        Eggs
        Herring, cod ovary
        Wheat germ, bran, dried peas, peanuts
        Yeast, royal jelly
    Medium: 0.5 mg-2.0 mg/100 g
        Salmon, clams, mackerel
        Walnuts
        Broccoli, soybeans, oats, lima beans, cauliflower, peas, avocado, carrots, kale, dried lentils, spinach, rice
        Beef, pork (ham, bacon), chicken, lamb
        Mushrooms, wheat, cheese
    Low: 0.1-0.5 mg/100 g
        Bananas, oranges, peaches, pears, pineapples, tomatoes, apples, grapes, grapefruit, lemons, plums
        Onions, kidney beans, cabbage, lettuce, peppers, white and sweet potatoes, turnips, watercress
        Almonds
        Oysters, lobster, shrimp
        Veal
        Milk, honey, molasses

MEDICAL AND NUTRITIONAL ROLE

1. **Units:** By weight, mg

2. **Normal Blood Levels:** 19-32 μg/100 ml

3. **Recommended Allowances**
    Children—no data
    Adults—Exact values unknown, estimate 10-15 mg/day
    Special—Increased needs in stress situations

4. **Administration**
    Injection—Parenteral
    Topical—No data
    Oral—Preferred route

5. **Factors Affecting Availability**
    Decrease
        Cooking—Up to 44% loss
        Heat instability
        Difficult release of bound forms
    Increase: Intestinal bacteria synthesis (very little in man)

6. **Deficiency Symptoms**
    General
        Neuromotor disturbances
        Cardiovascular disorders
        Digestive disorders
        Infection susceptibility
        Physical weakness, depression
    Stress susceptibility—rats
    Skin disorders (cornea)—rats, chicks
    Liver disorder—rat, chick
    Reproductive failure—chick
    Decreased antibody production—rat

7. **Effects of Overdose**
    10 g/kg in mice, respiratory failure
    Essentially nontoxic in man

METABOLIC ROLE

1. **Biosynthesis**
    Precursors
        α-Ketoisovaleric acid (pantoic acid)
        Uracil (β-alanine)
        Aspartic acid (β-alanine)
    Intermediates
        Ketopantoic cid
        Pantoic acid
        β-alanine

2. **Production: Species and Sites**
    Plants—Green plants, fungi
    Bacteria—Intestinal

3. **Storage:** Possibly liver, heart, kidney (all small amounts)

4. **Blood Carriers:**   Blood proteins

5. **Half-life:**   Estimate average loss: 25% of daily requirements

6. **Target tissues:**   All, esp. brain, heart, kidney, liver

7. **Reactions**
   Coenzyme form: CoA (adenine -3′-P-Ribose-P-P-pantothenic acid-β-mercapto ethylamine)

Organ	Enzyme System	Effect
Liver	TRANSFERASE: Citrate condensing enzyme β-Ketothiolase, CoA transferase	Activated
Brain	TRANSACYLASES: Choline acetylase, lipoic transacetylase, phosphotransacetylase	Activated
Liver	ISOMERASES: Methylmalonyl isomerase, β-hydroxyacyl racemase, enoyl isomerase	Activated
Liver	ESTERASES: Acetyl CoA deacylase, succinyl CoA deacylase	Activated
Liver	HYDRASES: Enoylhydrase	Activated
Liver	SYNTHETASES: Acetic thiokinase, fatty acid thiokinases, succinic thiokinase, acetyl carboxylase, propionyl carboxylase, methyl crotonylcarboxylase	Activated
Muscle and liver	DEHYDROGENASES: Hydroxyacyldehydrogenase, pyruvate dehydrogenase, α-ketoglutarate dehydrogenase acyl dehydrogenases	Activated

8. **Mode of Action**
   Cellular
   Anabolic
   Lipid synthesis increased
   Active in synthesis of porphyrins, acetylcholine and isoprenoid groups
   Sterol and hormone synthesis increased
   Catabolic—Regulates CHO metabolism
   Other—As coenzyme A in CHO, lipid, and protein metabolism. Acyl transfer agent.
   Organismal
   Fat synthesis and breakdown
   Respiratory pigment synthesis
   Water metabolism regulator
   Energy metabolism regulator

9. **Catabolism**
   Intermediates—Not destroyed in body
   Excretion Products
      Urine—Pantothenic acid (1-7 mg/day)
      Feces—Variable

MISCELLANEOUS

1. **Relationship to Other Vitamins**
   Folic acid—Required for utilization of pantothenic acid
   Biotin—Required for utilization of pantothenic acid; acts with panto-
      thenic acid in fatty acid biosynthesis; reduces severity of panto-
      thenic acid deficiency in rats
   Vitamin C—Compensates partly for deficiency of pantothenic acid
   CoQ—Decreased in pantothenic acid deficiency
   Vitamin A and Vitamin E—Synthesis promoted by pantothenic acid
      (isoprene production)
   Pantothenic acid and biotin involved in synthesis of niacin

2. **Relationship to Hormones**
   Aldosterone, Deoxycorticosterone, Cortisol, Testosterone, Progeste-
      rone—Cholesterol precursors for sterol hormones in adrenal cortex
      require pantothenic acid for synthesis; pantothenic acid deficiency
      produces cortical necrosis
   Cortisone—Relieves certain pantothenic acid deficiency symptoms in
      humans
   STH—Produces pantothenic acid deficiency in rats; synergist in growth

3. **Unusual Features**
   Promotes amino acid uptake
   Anticarcinogenic agent (?) (A. E. Needham)
   Potentiated by Zn in preventing graying of hair in rats
   Resistance to stress of cold immersion
   Deficiency of pantothenic acid in tumors
   Chick hatchability depends on pantothenic acid
   Useful in treating vertigo, postoperative shock, poisoning with isoniazid
      and curare
   Useful in acceleration of wound healing
   Useful in treating Addison's disease, liver cirrhosis, and diabetes

4. Possible Relationships of Deficiency Symptoms to Metabolic Action

Neuromotor Disturbances

Decreased phospholipid and acetylcholine synthesis

Has effect on membranes, degeneration of nerves

Cardiovascular disorders—Disturbances of fat and CHO metabolism due to degeneration of liver

Digestive disorders—Decreased bile acid production due to decreased sterol production; atrophy of intestinal mucosa

Infection susceptibility—Decreased antibody production due to decreased ATP synthesis

Physical weakness and depression—Decreased ATP synthesis

16
Hypothalamic-
Releasing Factors

CORTICOTROP(H)IN-RELEASING HORMONE (CRH)

1. **Synonyms:** CRF, cortical-releasing factor (hormone), (adreno) corti-cotrop(h)in-releasing factor

2. **History**
   1955—Saffran *et al.* first demonstrated release of ACTH by crude hypothalamic extract
   1962—Schally *et al.* proposed structure for CRH
   1963—Critchlow *et al.* reported CRH preparation maintains ACTH synthesis in pituitary transplants

3. **Forms:** α_1, α_2, and β

4. **Analogs:** Vasopressin, oxytocin

5. **Functions:** Chemical stimulant; messenger from hypothalamus to ACTH-producing cells in anterior pituitary; stimulates production of ACTH

6. **Structure**
   Peptide with disulfide ring system
   α_1—16 amino acids, similar to α-MSH
   α_2—13 amino acids, almost identical to α-MSH
   β—11 amino acids, similar to arginine vasopressin

7. MW—Approx. 1100 (β), 1500 (α)

8. **Extraction; Purification:**   Acid acetone, pH 1.5, ppt. with $(NH_4)_2SO_4$, chromatography, countercurrent distribution

9. **Determination**
   Bioassay—Release of corticosteroids in rat plasma on injection of CRH

10. **Factors Affecting Release of CRH**
    Stimulators—Stress, low level of cortisol, sympathomimetic amines
    Inhibitors—Cerebral cortex factors

11. **Production Sites and Storage Location**
    Hypothalamus—Ventral area, neurohypophysis

12. **Target Tissues:**   Anterior pituitary (ACTH-producing cells)

13. **Reactive Intermediate:**   Cyclic AMP

14. **Unusual Features:**   Very unstable

LUTEINIZING HORMONE-RELEASING HORMONE (LRH)

1. **Synonyms:**   LRF, LH-releasing factor (hormone)

2. **History**
   1941—Guillemin first postulated existence of LH-releasing factor
   1964—McCann and Ramirez caused depletion of ovarian ascorbic acid with extracts of hypothalamus
   1964—Campbell *et al.* infused hypothalamic extract into anterior pituitary and produced ovulation

3. **Functions:**   Chemical stimulant: messenger from hypothalamus to LH-producing cells in anterior pituitary

4. **Structure:**   Peptide containing Asp., Glu., Gly., Ala., Lys., His., Arg., Thr., Prol., Leu., Ser.

5. MW—1200-2500

6. **Extraction; Purification:**   Acetic acid extraction; gel filtration on sephadex G-25, chromatography

7. **Determination:**   Bioassay—Depletion of ovarian vit. C

8. **Factors Affecting Release of LRH**
   Stimulators—Low levels of estradiol, testosterone, norepinephrine, cate-
      cholamines
   Inhibitors—High levels of LH, testosterone

9. **Production Sites and Storage Location:**   Hypothalamus

10. **Target Tissues:**   Anterior pituitary (LH-producing cells)

11. **Reactive Intermediate:**   Cyclic AMP

THYROTROP(H)IN-RELEASING HORMONE (TRH)

1. **Synonyms:**   TRF, TSH-releasing factor (hormone)

2. **Antagonists:**   T3, T4 (large doses)

3. **History**
   1958—Harris and Woods produced thyroidal I_{131} release on stimulation
      of hypothalamus
   1958—Nikitovich *et al.* produced TSH after reimplanting pituitary graft
      near median eminence, but not in temporal lobe area
   1969—Byler *et al.* determined structure of porcine TRH

4. **Functions:**   Chemical stimulant: messenger from hypothalamus to TSH-
      producing cells in anterior pituitary

5. **Structure:**   Porcine TRH: Tripeptide
   L-pyroglutamyl—L-histidyl—L-proline amide

6. **MW:**   Approx. 400

7. **Extraction: Purification:**   Gel filtration; high-voltage electrophoresis

8. **Factors Affecting Release of TRH**
   Stimulators—Low level of T4, cold, stress, light, Ca^{++} ion
   Inhibitors—No data

9. **Production Sites and Storage Location:**   Suprachiasmatic area, median
      eminence, neurohypophysis

10. **Target Tissue:**   Anterior pituitary (TSH-producing cells)

11. **Reactive Intermediate:**   Cyclic AMP

12. **Unusual Properties:**   Destroyed in human serum in 15 min at 37° C

FOLLICLE STIMULATING HORMONE-RELEASING HORMONE (FRH)

1. **Synonyms:**   FSH-RF, FSH-releasing factor (hormone), FRF, FSH-RH

2. **History**
   1932—Hollweg and Junkmann proposed CNS involved in secretion of gonadotropins
   1964—Igarishi *et al.* demonstrated FSH-releasing activity of hypothalamic extracts
   1964—Mittler and Meites demonstrated FRH increases release of FSH in pituitary culture

3. **Functions:**   Chemical stimulant: messenger from hypothalamus to FSH-producing cells in anterior pituitary

4. **Structure:**   Polyamine, MW = < 300

5. **Extraction: Purification:**   Similar to LRH, plus long columns of sephadex G-25.

6. **Factors Affecting Release of FRH**
   Stimulators—Estrogen level (cyclic), K^+ ion
   Inhibitors—Stress, FSH

7. **Production Sites and Storage Location:**   Median eminence

8. **Target Tissues:**   Anterior pituitary (FSH-producing cells)

9. **Reactive Intermediate:**   Cyclic AMP

PROLACTIN RELEASE-INHIBITING HORMONE (PIH)

1. **Synonyms:**   PIF, RIH, prolactin inhibiting factor (hormone)

2. **History**
     1963—Meites showed increased prolactin secretion by pituitaries in tissue culture while other hormones decreased
     1962-63—Talwalker; Basteels *et al.* reduced prolactin in pituitary culture by adding hypothalamic extract

3. **Functions:** Chemical inhibitor: messenger from hypothalamus to prolactin-producing cells in anterior pituitary

4. **Structure:**   Some similarity to LRH, probably a peptide

5. **Extraction: Purification:**   0.1 *N* HCl extract, concentrate and separate on sephadex G-25

6. **Factors Affecting Release of PIH**
     Stimulator—Prolactin
     Inhibitor—Reserpine

7. **Production Sites and Storage Location:**   Satiety center, appetite suppressor in hypothalamus

8. **Target Tissues:**   Prolactin-producing cells in anterior pituitary

9. **Reactive Forms:**   No data

10. **Unusual Features:**   Stable to boiling

GROWTH HORMONE-RELEASING HORMONE (GRH)

1. **Synonyms:**   GRF, somatotrop(h)in-releasing factor (hormone), growth-hormone-releasing factor (hormone), SRF, GHRF

2. **History**
     1964—Deuben and Meites released GH in rat pituitary in tissue culture using rat hypothalamic extracts
     1965—Schally *et al.* stimulated release of GH by incubating rat pituitaries with beef, pig, hypothalamic extracts

3. **Functions:**   Chemical stimulant; messenger from hypothalamus to STH-producing cells in anterior pituitary

4. **Structure:**   Acidic polypeptide

5. **MW:**   2500 (approx.)

6. **Extraction: Purification:**   0.1 N HCl extraction; gel filtration, CMC chromatography

7. **Factors Affecting Release of GRH**
   Stimulators—No data
   Inhibitors—No data

8. **Production Sites and Storage Location:**   Hypothalamus, neurohypophysis

9. **Target Tissues:**   Anterior pituitary cells producing STH

10. **Reactive Intermediate:**   Cyclic AMP

PROLACTIN-RELEASING HORMONE (PRH)

1. **Synonyms:**   PRF, prolactin-releasing factor (hormone)

2. **History**
   1965—Kragt and Meites increased prolactin release in pigeon pituitary culture by pigeon hypothalamic extracts

3. **Functions:**   Stimulates release of prolactin from anterior pituitary (probably only in birds)

4. **Structure:**   Not obtained pure

5. **Extraction: Purification:**   No data

6. **Factors Affecting Release of PRH**
   Stimulators—No data
   Inhibitors—No data

7. **Production Sites and Storage Location:**   Hypothalamus of birds

8. **Target Tissues:**   Anterior pituitary cells secreting prolactin

MELANOCYTE STIMULATING HORMONE RELEASE-INHIBITING HORMONE (MIH)

1. **Synonyms:** MIF, MSH-inhibiting factor (hormone), MRIH

2. **History**
   1962—Etkin produced frog blackening by repositioning pituitary in other locations in body
   1964—Kastin and Ross produced coloration in albino rat by repositioning pituitary

3. **Functions:** Inhibits release of MSH from intermediate lobe of pituitary

4. **Structure:** Not obtained pure

5. **Extraction: Purification:** 2 N acetic acid extraction; gel filtration on sephadex G-25

6. **Factors Affecting Release of MIH**
   Stimulators—No data
   Inhibitors—No data

7. **Production Sites and Storage Location:** Hypothalamus (paraventricular nucleus)

8. **Target Tissues:** Cells of intermediate pituitary lobe secreting MSH

MELANOCYTE STIMULATING HORMONE-RELEASING HORMONE (MRH)

1. **Synonyms:** MRH, MSH-releasing factor (hormone)

2. **History**
   1965—Taliesnik and Orios found evidence for existence of MRH

3. **Functions:** Stimulates release of MSH from intermediate lobe of pituitary

4. **Structure:** Not obtained pure

5. **Extraction: Purification:** No data

6. Factors Affecting Release of MRH
    Stimulators: No data
    Inhibitors: No data

7. Production Sites and Storage Location: No data

8. Target Tissues: Cells of intermediate pituitary lobe secreting MSH

17
Growth Hormone

GENERAL INFORMATION

1. **Synonyms:** Somatotrop(h)in, GH, STH, phyone, (anterior) pituitary growth hormone, adenohypophyseal growth hormone, somatotrophic hormone, hypophyseal growth hormone

2. **History**
   - 1921—Evans and Long induced growth in rats with pituitary extract
   - 1930—Smith restored growth in hypophysectomized rats with hypophyseal implants
   - 1945—Li *et al.* isolated growth hormone from anterior pituitary (beef)
   - 1962—Reisfeld *et al.* isolated growth hormone from human anterior pituitary
   - 1964—Glick, Roth, Berson, and Yalow developed accurate immunoassay of growth hormone in serum
   - 1966—Li *et al.* determined amino acid sequence for human growth hormone, 188 amino acid residues
   - 1971—Li *et al.* synthesized human growth hormone

3. **Physiological Forms:** "Sulfation factor"

4. **Active Analogs and Related Forms:** Prolactin (human). Chorionic factor

5. **Inactive Analogs and Related Forms:** Primate GH minus 10% A.A. residues, bovine GH minus 25% A.A.'s, human GH minus C-terminal phenylalanine

6. **Antagonists:**   Cortisone, cortisol, insulin (all concentration dependent), plasma inhibitors

7. **Synergists:**   Adrenal corticoids (fat metabolism), ACTH, T4, insulin, testosterone

8. **Physiological Functions**
   General growth of organism
   Promotes skeletal growth, protein anabolism, fat metabolism, CHO metabolism, water and salt metabolism

9. **Deficiency Diseases and Disorders**
   Deficiency—Progeria, pituitary dwarf, hypopituitarism
   Excess—Acromegaly, gigantism

10. **Essentiality for Life:**   Absence results in stunted, abnormal growth, with possible decrease in normal lifespan

CHEMISTRY

1. **Structure**—Growth hormone, structure known and synthesized (Human)
   Human—Coiled, unbranched protein, 188 A.A. residues, 2S-S-bridges
   (Phe ———— Phe)
   Bovine—Coiled, 1-branch protein, 400 A.A. residues, 4S-S-bridges

   Phe`⁻⁻`~~~> Phe
   Ala`⁻⁻⁻⁻`

2. **Reactions**

Heat—Stable to 100°C 15 min	Oxidation—Oxidizes S—S bonds
Acid—Unstable (strong)	Reduction—Reduces S—S bonds
Alkali—Unstable (strong)	Light—No data
Water—Soluble, acidic	Proteolysis—15% limit of digestion of human growth hormone before loses activity

3. **Properties**

Appearance—No data	Solubility
MW—21,500 (human)	H_2O—Sol.
48,000 (bovine)	Acet. Alc.—Insol.
MP—None	Benz., Chl., Eth.—Insol.
Crystal Form—None	Absn. Max.—Approx. 280 mμ
Salts—None	Chemical Nature—Simple protein, globulin
Important Groups for activity	Misc- pI = 4.9 (human)
—S—S—; Phe (terminal)	= 6.8 (bovine)

4. **Commercial Production:**   Not available

5. **Isolation**

Sources—Pituitary glands of sheep, ox, pig, monkey
Methods
Extract with borate buffer, pH 8.8, DEAE chromatography
Ppt. with $(NH_4)_2SO_4$, column chromatog. IRC_5O, pH 5.1
Treat with acetic acid-acet., ppt. with acet.; column chromatog., ppt. with alc.
Additional purification: Counter-current distribution and gel filtration

6. **Determination**

Bioassay
Tibia test (rat) (5 μg-120 μg)
Increased weight (rat)
Increased N retention (rat)
S^{35} incorporation into cartilage (rat)
Physicochemical
Immunoassay
Radioimmunoassay

MEDICAL AND BIOLOGICAL ROLE

1. **Species Occurrence, Specificity and Antigenicity**

Occurrence—All vertebrates except birds
Specificity—No crossing of species lines for primates or guinea pigs. Other vertebrates slightly more tolerant
Antigenicity—Monkey, sheep, rat, pig hormones antigenically different.

2. **Units:**   1 USP unit = 1 I.U. = 1 mg

3. **Normal Blood Levels:**   20-50 μg/100 ml serum (man)

4. **Administration**

Injection—Preferred route
Topical—Not used
Oral—Not used, inactivated

5. **Factors Affecting Release**

Inhibitors—Inadequate dietary protein, sleeplessness, hyperglycemia
Stimulators—Plasma amino acids, hypoglycemia, GHRH, vasopressin (fish), adequate protein in diet, fasting, exercise, sleep

6. **Deficiency Symptoms**
    Humans
        Dwarfism
        Failure of long bones to close
        Failure of sexual maturation
        Increased fat deposition

7. **Effects of Overdose, Excess**
    Tumors, β-cell destruction
    Pituitary giants
    Bone thickening

METABOLIC ROLE

1. **Biosynthesis**
    Precursors—Amino acids. All 20 standard
    Intermediates—Unknown
    Site(s) in Cell—Unknown

2. **Production Sites:** Anterior pituitary acidophils

3. **Storage Areas:** Anterior pituitary

4. **Blood Carriers:** α_2-Macroglobulin, β-lipoprotein

5. **Half-life:** 20 min

6. **Target Tissues:** All except nervous tissue, esp. bone, viscera, muscle, epiphyseal cartilage

7. **Reactions**
    Reactive form—Sulfation factor (?)

Organ	Enzyme System	Effect
Most tissues and organs	RNA-polymerase	Activated
	Protein-synthetic	Activated
Blood cells	Alk. phosphatase	Activated

8. **Mode of Action**
    Cellular
        Anabolic
            Increases rate of protein and RNA synthesis
            Increases glycogen deposition (muscles)

Catabolic—Mobilizes unsaturated fatty acids

Other—Increases amino acid permeability of cells; increases salt and H_2O transport in kidney

Organismal

Increases muscle, skin, viscera, lymph glands, bone and cartilage size

Decreases urea formation

Increases blood sugar

Increases tissue nitrogen

Mobilizes fatty acids from adipose tissue

9. Catabolism

Intermediates—Liver destruction, to peptides; plasmin in blood inactivates GH

Excretion Products—Small amounts of GH in urine

MISCELLANEOUS

1. Relationship to Vitamins

All vitamins—All concerned with growth

2. Relationship to Other Hormones

Insulin—Inhibited by GH in certain concentrations. Synergist with GH at other (low) concentrations

GHR—GH-releasing factor of hypothalamus

Vasopressin—A hypothalamic release factor (in fish)

Cortisol—Antagonist to GH (protein metabolism). Also a synergist (fat metabolism)

Testosterone—Synergist with GH

T4—Synergist with GH (differentiation)

ACTH—Synergist with GH

3. Unusual Features

Rat GH lacks tryptophan; contaminated with protease

Lactogenic and growth activity present in human GH

Guinea pig not sensitive to own GH

HGH withstands 15 min at $100°C$

Increases capacity to form tumors

Lactogenic action in humans, similarity in structure to prolactin

4. **Possible Relationships of Deficiency Symptoms to Metabolic Action**

Dwarfism—Lack of protein synthesis due to lack of GH activity

Failure of long bones to close—Lack of major metabolic action of GH

Failure of sexual maturation—Lack of synergism of sex hormones and GH

Increased fat deposition—Lack of catabolic action of GH

18
Thyroid-Stimulating Hormone (TSH)

GENERAL INFORMATION

1. **Synonyms:** Thyroid-stimulating hormone, thyr(e)otrop(h)ic hormone, TTH, thyrotrop(h)in

2. **History**

   1921—Evans and Long first noted effects of pituitary extracts on growth

   1927-30—Smith reported that hypophysectomy in rat causes atrophy of thyroids (and other organs) correctable by hypophyseal implants

   1929—Basset; Aron and Loeb defined properties of a thyrotrophic hormone

   1945—Ciereszko isolated crude TSH from beef pituitaries

   1960—Wynston et al. obtained purified TSH from beef, sheep, and whale pituitaries

   1963—Carsten et al. determined amino acid composition of beef TSH

3. **Physiological Forms:** Unknown

4. **Active Analogs and Related Compounds:** LATS (long-acting thyroid stimulator)

5. **Inactive Analogs and Related Compounds:** TSH minus CHO moeity, oxidized TSH

6. **Antagonists:** Acetylated TSH, p-aminosalicylic acid, perchlorate, sulfathiazole, thiocyanate, thiouracil, thiourea

7. **Synergists:** STH, ACTH, MSH, TH

8. **Physiological Functions**
    Regulation of body temperature via T4
    Maintains thyroid gland and its secretory activity (colloid discharge)
    Maintains iodine uptake by thyroid gland
    Promotes differentiation in embryo during development (via T4)
    Stimulates coupling of diiodotyrosine to form thyroxine (T4)

9. **Deficiency Diseases, Disorders**
    Thyrotoxicosis (excess), goiter (excess or deficiency), exophthalmos (excess), Sheehan's syndrome (deficiency)

10. **Essentiality for Life:**   Required by all vertebrates for proper development; possible shortening of lifespan in absence of TSH

CHEMISTRY

1. **Structure**
    Glycoprotein—Unpurified (contaminated with LH). Contains 2.5% CHO—Glucosamine, galactosamine, hexose, fucose

2. **Reactions**

    Heat—Inactivates
    Acid—Easily inactivates
    Alkali—Inactivates
    Water Basic

    Oxidation—Inactivates using bromine, iodine, and permanganate
    Reduction—May potentiate effects of TSH
    Light—No data
    Proteolysis—inactivates with pepsin or trypsin

3. **Properties**

    Appearance—No data
    MW—26-30,000 (300 amino acids)
    MP—No data
    Crystal Form—No data
    Salts—No data
    Important Groups for activity
        α-NH$_2$, tyrosine, CHO moiety
        —S—S—

    Solubility
        H_2O—Sol.
        Acet., Alc.—Insol.
        Benz., Chl., Eth.—Insol.
    Absn. Max.—Approx 280 mμ
    Chemical Nature—Basic glycoprotein, globulin
    MISC—pI = 7·8

4. **Commercial Production:**   Extract bovine pituitary glands

5. **Isolation**
   Sources—Bovine pituitary glands
   Methods
       Extract pituitary (freeze, dried) in 2% NaCl, pH 7.6. Precipitate at pI
           with acetone (1 I.U./mg)
       Precipitate from 3.6 M ammonium sulfate
   Purification
       Chromatog. on IRC-50, elute with 1 M NaCl
       Chromatog. on CM cell, elute with 0.2 M NaCl 0.05 M formate, pH
           3-4
       Gel filtration on sephadex G-50, G-100
       Chromatog. on IRC-50 in urea (60 I.U./mg)

6. **Determination**
   Bioassay
       Height of secretory epithelium in thyroid—guinea pig
       Number colloid droplets in guinea pig thyroid
       I_2 depletion of 1-day chick
       Uptake I^{131} by thyroid of rats
       In vitro assay, slice uptake of I^{131}
   Physicochemical—Radioimmunoassay

MEDICAL AND BIOLOGICAL ROLE

1. **Species Occurrence, Specificity, and Antigenicity**
   Occurrence—All vertebrates
   Specificity—Incomplete; bovine TSH active in all species
       (chick and guinea pig most sensitive)
   Antigenicity—High; bovine TSH antigenic in rabbits

2. **Units:**   1 I.U. = 13.5 mg of standard = 1 USP unit

3. **Normal Blood Levels (Man):**   5-20 milliunits/100 ml plasma

4. **Administration**
   Injection—Preferred route
   Topical—Inactive
   Oral—Inactive

5. **Factors Affecting Release**
   Inhibitors
      Feedback via hypothalamus from high serum T4
      High serum iodide, massive doses vit. A
      High temperature
      Inhibition of hypothalamus
      Nerve stimuli
   Stimulators
      Release factor of hypothalamus (TRH)
      Decreased serum T4 via hypothalamus
      Low temperature
      Stimulation of hypothalamus
      Nerve stimuli

6. **Deficiency Symptoms**
   Decreased synthesis of thyroid hormones
   Low serum protein-bound iodine (PBI)
   Decreased iodine uptake by thyroid
   Secondary symptoms of thyroxine deficiency

7. **Effects of Overdose, Excess**
   Exophthalmic effect
   Increased synthesis of thyroid hormones
   Increased PBI
   Increased iodide uptake by thyroid
   Increased basal metabolic rate
   Decreased thyroid iodine
   Decreased blood cholesterol
   Goiter

METABOLIC ROLE

1. **Biosynthesis**
   Precursors—17 of 20 standard amino acids. No glutamine, asparagine,
      tryptophan
   Intermediates—Unknown
   Site(s) in cell—Basophilic cytoplasm

2. **Production Sites:** S^2 type cell, anterior pituitary

3. **Storage Areas:**   Not stored

4. **Blood Carriers:** β-globulins

5. **Half-life:**   54 min

6. **Target Tissues:**   Thyroid, reproductive glands, liver, probably muscles

7. **Reactions**
    Reactive intermediate—Cyclic AMP (secondary messenger)

Organ	Enzyme System	Effect
Thyroid	Proteolytic enzymes (on colloid)	Activated
Thyroid	Synthetic enzymes for T4	Activated
Thyroid	Adenyl cyclase	Activated
Thyroid	DPN kinase	Activated
Thyroid	HMP enzymes	Activated

8. **Mode of Action**
    Cellular
        Anabolic
            RNA and protein synthesis (thyroid)
            Thyroid hormone synthesis (thyroid)
        Catabolic
            Lipolytic activity increased
            Proteolytic activity increased (thyroid)
            Glucose oxidation increased via TCA, HMP, and glycolysis
        Other
            Activates thyroid cell membrane enzymes
            Increases oxidase granules (thyroid), and O_2 consumption by thyroid cells
            Increases glucose and iodine entry into cells
            No increase in $NADP^+$
    Organismal
        Mobilization of thyroid hormones
        Increases serum bound iodine
        Maintains body temperature via T4

9. **Catabolism**
    Intermediates—Hydrolyzed in liver
    Excretion products—Present in urine

MISCELLANEOUS

1. Relationship to Vitamins

Vitamin A—Massive doses of vit. A inhibit secretion of TSH; thyroid hormones required for carotene and retinene conversions

Vitamins B_1, B_2, B_{12}, C—Requirements increased in hyperthyroidism; tissue concentrations reduced

Vitamin B_6, Niacin—Conversion to phosphorylated reactive forms impaired in hyperthyroidism

Vitamins A, D, E, K—Requirements increased in hyperthyroidism; tissue concentrations reduced in hyperthyroidism

2. Relationship to Other Hormones

T4—TSH stimulates production of T4; synergist in lactation

LH—Contained frequently as a contaminant in TSH

3. Unusual Features

Not inactivated by neuraminidase

CHO moiety needed for activity

Different functions in lower species

Rapid loss of potency in solution

Inactivation by freeze drying

Reduction may potentiate activity

High cystine content

Phospholipase activity of TSH reported

4. Possible Relationships of Deficiency Symptoms to Metabolic Action

Decreased synthesis of thyroid hormones—Insufficient activation of thyroid cell membrane enzymes

Low serum PBI—Reduction of T4 output due to decreased TSH

Decreased iodide uptake by thyroid—Decreased reactivity of thyroid gland

19
Follicle-
Stimulating
Hormone (FSH)

GENERAL INFORMATION

1. **Synonyms:** Follotropin, Luteoantine, Thylakentrin, Prolan A, gonadotropin I, gametogenic hormone, follicle ripening hormone, gameto-
   kinetic hormone

2. **History**
   - 1921—Evans and Long first noted gonadotropic effect of pituitary
     extracts on rats
   - 1927-30—Smith reported that hypophysectomy in rat causes atrophy of
     gonads (and other organs) correctable by hypophyseal im-
     plants
   - 1928—Aschheim and Zondek discovered a follicle-stimulating gona-
     dotropin in menopausal urine
   - 1933—Fevold *et al.* identified a separate follicle-stimulating hormone in
     the pituitary
   - 1939—Chow *et al.* demonstrated FSH to be resistant to inactivation by
     proteolytic enzymes
   - 1940—Fevold *et al.*   } Described isolation procedures
   - 1949—Li, Simpson and Evans } for animal FSH
   - 1965—Roos and Gemzell prepared human FSH from menopausal urine

3. **Physiological Forms:** Unknown

4. **Active Analogs and Related Forms:** PMSG, HMG (mixture of FSH and
   LH)

5. **Inactive Analogs and Related Forms:**   FSH without sialic acid moiety

6. **Antagonists:**   No data

7. **Synergists:**   LH, STH, T4

8. **Physiological Functions:**   Gametogenic
   Female—Stimulates ovarian follicles to grow and to develop, forming multiple layers and antra
   Male—Stimulates seminiferous tubules; stimulates spermatogenesis

9. **Deficiency Diseases, Disorders:**   Klinefelter's syndrome (deficiency), Turner's syndrome (deficiency), hypogonadotropic eunochoidism (deficiency)

10. **Essentiality for Life:**   Not required for life of organism, but required for reproduction by all vertebrates analyzed

CHEMISTRY

1. **Structure:**   Unknown
   Glycoprotein—7.4% sialic acid; impure preparations (contam. with LH) 0.6% hexosamine; 1.3% hexose

2. **Reactions**

   Heat—No data
   Acid—Stable
   Alkali—Stable
   Water—Acidic

   Oxidation—H_2O_2, periodate
   —inactivate
   Reduction—Cysteine, ketene—inactivate
   Light—No data
   Proteolysis—Inactivates on 60-75% digestion with trypsin
   Urea—Stable in 6 M urea

3. **Properties**

   Appearance—No data
   MW—30,000 (pig)
   28,000 (sheep)
   MP—No data
   Crystal Form—No data
   Salts—No data

   Important Groups for activity
   Sialic acid (complex CHO)
   —S—S—, terminal NH_2
   Solubility
   H_2O—soluble
   Acet., Alc.—Insol.
   Sol. 50% Acet.

Sol. 70% Alc.   Misc—pI = 5.1 (pig)
Benz., Chl., Eth.—Insol.   = 4.5 (sheep)
Absn. Max.—Approx 280 mμ
Chemical Nature—Acidic
glycoprotein

4. **Commercial Production:**   Extracted from human and sheep pituitaries

5. **Isolation**
Sources—Human, horse, sheep, swine pituitary
Method—Extract frozen pituitaries in aqueous salts; fractional precipitation from ammonium sulfate; DEAE cellulose; sephadex G-100;
polyacrylamide gel electrophoresis

6. **Determination**
Bioassay—Problems with LH contamination
Ovarian weight change
Stimulation of young ovarian follicles (rabbit)
Increase in weight of testes
Physiochemical
Immunoassay
Radioimmunassay

MEDICAL AND BIOLOGICAL ROLE

1. **Species, Occurrence, Specificity, and Antigenicity**
Occurrence—Found in all species of vertebrates studied
Specificity—Strong species specificity (Fish FSH inactive in mammals)
Antigenicity—Moderately antigenic

2. **Units:**   1 I.U. = 38.5 μg sheep FSH (NIH—S_1, Std.)

3. **Normal Blood Levels (Man):**   Males: 0.02 I.U./100 ml plasma, females
0.015 I.U./100 ml plasma (Menopausal female: 0.20 I.U./100 ml
plasma)

4. **Administration**
Injection—Preferred route
Topical—inactive
Oral—inactive

5. **Factors Affecting Release**
   Inhibitors—Estradiol, cortisol, stress, hyperthyroidism, feedback by sex hormones via hypothalamus
   Stimulators—FRH from hypothalamus, castration, menopause, low sex hormone levels, female—rhythmic control by hypothalamus via FRH secretion, male—continuous secretion of FRH by hypothalamus

6. **Deficiency Symptoms**
   Decreased gametogenic function and development (nonfunctional)
   Atrophy of gonads
   No maturation of ova, sperm
   Obesity
   Decreased libido, potency, hair growth
   Decreased blood levels of estrogen

7. **Effects of Overdose, Excess**
   Hypertrophy of secondary sex organs
   Increased growth and maturation of numerous follicles
   Increased estrogen secretion (with LH)
   Follicular cysts

METABOLIC ROLE

1. **Biosynthesis**
   Precursors—All 20 standard amino acids except methionine
   Intermediates—Unknown

2. **Production Sites:**   Anterior pituitary—basophilic cells (peripheral)

3. **Storage Areas:**   Anterior pituitary

4. **Blood Carriers:** α, β-plasma proteins

5. **Half-Life:**   Approx. 1 hr

6. **Target Tissues:**   Ovary, testis

7. **Reactions**
   Reactive Form—Unknown
   Enzyme Systems—Unknown

8. **Mode of Action**
   Cellular
      Anabolic—Unknown
      Catabolic—Unknown
      Other—Stimulates incorporation of glucose and α-aminoisobutyric acid into rat ovaries
   Organismal
      Promotes growth of ovarian follicles
      Promotes development of ovarian follicle
      Promotes growth of seminiferous tubules
      Promotes spermatogenesis

9. **Catabolism**
   Intermediates—Liver hydrolysis
   Excretion Products—Free in urine (active)—small amounts

MISCELLANEOUS

1. **Relationship to Vitamins**
   Vitamin C—Depletion in ovary due to LH and FSH action
   Vitamin E—Needed for maintenance of membranes in sex organs

2. **Relationship to Other Hormones**
   STH, LH—Synergists to FSH
   PMSG, HMG—Active analogs to FSH
   ACTH—Inhibitor of FSH
   T4—Inhibitor of FSH

3. **Unusual Features**
   Increased instability with purer preparations
   Only pituitary hormone not precipitated with 50% saturated $(NH_4)_2SO_4$
   Bird migration, ovulation, sex behavior controlled by FSH via light and temperature
   Gonadotropins of mammals stimulate thyroids of fish
   CHO groups needed for activity—neuraminidase inactivates
   Cyclic release in females (spontaneous ovulators)

4. **Possible Relationships of Deficiency Symptoms to Metabolic Action**
   Decreased gametogenesis and development of gonads, atrophy of gonads, no maturation of ova or sperm, decreased potency—lack of FSH function (unknown)

Obesity—Unknown
Decreased libido—decreased synergism with testosterone and LH
Decreased hair growth—decreased synergism with sex hormones and LH
Decreased blood levels of estrogen—decreased synergism with LH

20
Luteinizing
Hormone (LH)

GENERAL INFORMATION

1. **Synonyms:** Luteotrop(h)in, interstitial cell-stimulating hormone, ICSH, Prolan B, gonadotrop(h)in II, Metakentrin, corpus luteum-ripening hormone

2. **History**
   1921—Evans and Long first noted gonadotropic effect of pituitary extracts on rats.
   1927-30—Smith noted hypophysectomy in rat caused atrophy of gonads (and other organs) correctable by hypophyseal implants
   1933—Fevold *et al.* identified a separate luteinizing hormone in pituitaries
   1940—Li, Simpson, and Evans isolated LH from sheep pituitaries
   1940—Shedlovsky *et al.* ⎫
   1942—Chow *et al.*   ⎬ Isolated LH from pig pituitaries
   1962—Squire *et al.* isolated a purified LH from human pituitaries

3. **Physiological Forms:** α and β-forms

4. **Active Analogs and Related Compounds**
   HCG, HMG (mixture of FSH and LH)
   PMSG (properties of FSH and LH)

5. **Inactive Analogs and Related Compounds:** LH minus CHO moiety

6. **Antagonists:**   Prolactin, insulin (both concentration dependent)

7. **Synergists:**   FSH, prolactin, TH, insulin

8. **Physiological Functions**
   Female
   Promotes estrogen and progesterone secretion, ovulation, maintains ovarian tissues
   Stimulates rupture of follicles and formation of corpora lutea
   Male
   Stimulates Leydig cells to secrete testosterone, gametogenic with FSH
   Promotes growth of seminal tubules and accessory sex organs

9. **Deficiency Diseases, Disorders:**   Hypogonadism; irregular sexual development

10. **Essentiality for Life:**   Not required for life of organism, but required for reproduction by all analyzed vertebrates

CHEMISTRY

1. **Structure**
   Globular glycoprotein with S—S bridges (2-5% CHO)
   Ser-Val-Asp———human
   Ser-Val-Phe———Ser-Lys (porcine)

2. **Reactions**

   Heat—Inactivates
   Acid—Picric, TCA, picrolonic, and flavianic acids ppt. LH without loss of activity
   Alkali—No data
   Water—Sol., acidic

   Oxidation—H_2O_2, periodate, performic acid—inactivate
   Reduction—Cysteine, ketene—inactivate
   Light—No data
   Proteolysis—Inactivates
   Urea—Unstable in 6 M urea

3. **Properties**

   Appearance—White powder
   MW—26,000 (human)
       30,000 (sheep)
   MP—No data
   Crystal Form—No data

   Salts—No data
   Important Groups for activity
     Cys., Pro.
     CHO moiety
     —S—S—

Solubility   Chemical Nature—Acidic, globular
  H_2O—soluble   glycoprotein
  Alc.—Sol. 4% alc.,   Misc—pI = 5.4 (human)
  Acet., Benz., Chl., Eth.—Insol.   = 7.3 (sheep)
  Absn. Max.—Approx 280 mμ = 7.45 (pig)

4. **Commercial Production:**   Extraction of human or sheep pituitaries

5. **Isolation**
 Sources—Pituitary of human, sheep, swine, and beef
 Method
  Aqueous extract at pH 5.5
  Ammonium sulfate precipitation
  Metaphosphoric acid precipitation
  Ethanol fractionation
  IRC-50; sephadex G-100

6. **Determination**
 Bioassay
  Vitamin C depletion of rat ovary
  Increased hyperemia in immature rat ovary
  Increased weight in male sex accessory organs
  Weaver-Finch test
  Physicochemical—Radioimmunoassay

MEDICAL AND BIOLOGICAL ROLE

1. **Species Occurrence, Specificity, and Antigenicity**
 Occurrence—Found in all vertebrate species studied
 Specificity—Slight species specificity
 Antigenicity—Definite

2. **Units:**   1 I.U. = 0.67 μg ovine LH (NIH—S$_1$, Std.)

3. **Normal Blood Levels (Man):**   1.5-3.0 I.U./100 ml plasma (males and females) preovulatory and menopausal women 7.5-15.0 I.U./100 ml plasma

4. **Administration**
 Injection—Preferred route
 Topical—Inactive
 Oral—Inactive

5. **Factors Affecting Release**
    Inhibitors
        Cortisol
        Stress
        High sex hormone levels
        Feedback to hypothalamus by sex hormones
        Hyperthyroidism
    Stimulators
        Low sex hormone levels
        External stimuli
        Male—Continuous LRH from hypothalamus
        Female—Continuous LRH (hypothalamus) in induced ovulators—rabbit
        Cyclic LRH (hypothalamus) in spontaneous ovulators—human and dog

6. **Deficiency Symptoms**
    Estrogen or androgen secretion inhibited
    Atrophy of interstitial tissue in ovary or testis
    Lack of ovulation, luteinization in female

7. **Effects of Overdose, Excess**
    Hypertrophy, then atrophy of Leydig cells in male
    Increases estrogen or androgen secretion (with FSH)
    Precocious ovulation and luteinization of prepared follicles

METABOLIC ROLE

1. **Biosynthesis**
    Precursors—19 of 20 standard amino acids, tryptophan missing
    Intermediates—Unknown

2. **Production Sites:**   Anterior pituitary, central cells, basophilic cells

3. **Storage Areas:**   Stored in pituitary prior to ovulation in female

4. **Blood Carriers:**   Complex with inactive protein

5. **Half-life:**   Approx. 1 hr

6. **Target Tissues:**   Gonads

7. Reactions
Reactive intermediate—Cyclic AMP (secondary messenger)

Organ	Enzyme System	Effect
Gonads	Adenyl cyclase	Activated
	Enzymes incorporating acetate into squalene	Activated

8. Mode of Action
Cellular
 Anabolic—Increased synthesis of steroid hormones
  Female—Interstitial ovarian cells synthesize estradiol
  Male—Leydig cells synthesize testosterone
 Catabolic—Increased CHO catabolism to produce NADH, NADP
Organismal
 Promotes gametogenesis
 Promotes growth of accessory sex organs
 Stimulates rupture of follicles in ovary

9. Catabolism
Intermediates—Hydrolysis in liver
Excretion products—Active hormone in urine

MISCELLANEOUS

1. Relationship to Vitamins
Vitamin C—Ovarian depletion on LH stimulation
Vitamin E—Involved in spermatogenesis

2. Relationship to Other Hormones
FSH—Synergist to LH
Prolactin—Synergist to LH
HMG—Mixture of FSH and LH
PMSG—Properties of FSH and LH
HCG—Analog to LH

3. Unusual Features
More stable on freeze-drying than FSH
LH causes multiple ovulation in birds
Insensitive to neuraminidase
Inactivated by trypsin and carboxypeptidase, pepsin, chymotrypsin

Not inactivated by CHO splitting enzymes; CHO moiety unharmed
CHO moiety needed for activity
Cyclic release in certain females (spontaneous ovulators)

4. **Possible Relationships of Deficiency Symptoms to Metabolic Action**
    Estrogen or androgen secretion inhibited—lack of cyclic AMP to stimulate ovary or testis production
    Atrophy of interstitial tissue in ovary or testis—lack of stimulus by cyclic AMP
    Lack of ovulation or luteinization in female—lack of cyclic AMP to initiate events leading to ovulation

21
Prolactin

GENERAL INFORMATION

1. **Synonyms:** Lactogenic hormone, luteotrop(h)ic hormone, LTH, luteotrop(h)in, lactogen, galactin, mammotropin

2. **History:**
   - 1928—Stricker and Grüter discovered prolactin
   - 1933—Riddle *et al.* coined term prolactin
   - 1937—Lyons isolated prolactin from pituitary glands of ox, sheep, and pig
   - 1939—Astwood, Fevold suggested luteotropin distinct from LH
   - 1941—Evans, Simpson, Lyons suggested identity of prolactin and luteotropin in rat
   - 1942—Li crystallized prolactin (first pituitary hormone to be crystallized)
   - 1967—Sherwood showed chemical similarity of human growth hormone to placental lactogenic hormone

3. **Physiological Forms:** In man, prolactin is a part of very pure growth hormone complex

4. **Active Analogs and Related Forms:** 50% digested residue—"active core"

5. **Inactive Analogs and Related Forms**
   - Reduced molecule (with cysteine)
   - Acetylated molecule—(on lysine residues)
   - Iodinated molecule—(tyrosine residues iodinated)

6. **Antagonists:** Progesterone, testosterone, estradiol, LH (all concentration dependent)

7. **Synergists:** STH, T4, prednisone, estradiol, progesterone, cortisol, oxytocin, PTH, LH

8. **Physiological Functions**
    Initiation of lactation
    Development of mammary glands in female
    Increases weight and growth (similar to somatotropin) (some species)
    Nidation of zygote
    Protein anabolism (some species)
    Growth and secretion of crop gland (birds)
    Luteotropic (only in mouse and rat)
    Promotes maternal behavior

9. **Deficiency Diseases, Disorders:** Mammary carcinoma, galactorrhea, failure of lactation

10. **Essentiality for Life:** Not essential except where it functions as a growth hormone in certain species (birds, reptiles)

CHEMISTRY

1. **Structure**
    Single chain protein, 205 amino acids
    Pig: Ala.———Cys—Tyr—Leu—Asn—Cys
    Sheep: Thre.———Cys—Tyr—Leu—Asn—Cys

2. **Reactions**

Heat—Stable	Oxidation—Inactivates
Acid—Ppt. with 0.5% TCA	Reduction—Inactivates
Alkali—Unstable	Light—Not reported
Water—Soluble, acidic	Proteolysis: 50% digestion leaves active core

3. **Properties**

Appearance—Crystalline powder	Salts—Not reported
MW—25,000 (pig)	Important Groups for activity
23,300 (sheep)	Tyr
MP—Not reported	Lys
Crystal Form—Not reported	Cys (S—S bridges)

Solubility:
H_2O—Slightly soluble
Alc.—Sol.
Acet., Benz., Chl., Ether—Insol.
Absn. Max.—Approx. 280 mμ

Chemical Nature—Single chain
simple acidic protein
$\alpha_D^{25} = -40.5°$ (H_2O)
Misc—pI = 4.97 (pig)
= 5.74 (sheep)

4. Commercial Production
Extraction of pituitary glands of ox, sheep, swine

5. Isolation
Sources—Pituitary glands of sheep
Methods
Ovine acetone powder extracted with pH 3 buffer
Precipitate prolactin with 0.06 saturated NaCl
Fractional precipitation, pH 5.6
Probability of protease contamination
Purify by: Countercurrent distribution. DEAE chromatography

6. Determination
Bioassay
Crop sac thickening (pigeons)
Mammary gland growth in pseudopregnant rabbit
Luteotropic, inhibition of estrus (mice)
Physicochemical Assay
Immunoassay
Radioimmunoassay

MEDICAL AND BIOLOGICAL ROLE

1. Species Occurrence, Specificity, and Antigenicity
Occurrence—Found in all vertebrates
Specificity—Some tolerance in crossing species lines
Antigenicity—Moderate; bovine X rabbit no antigenicity

2. Units: 1 I.U. = 0.1 mg international standard

3. Normal Blood Levels (Man)
Not detectable in male or nonlactating female
Detectable in lactating women

4. **Administration**
   Injection—Currently used
   Topical—Not active
   Oral—Not active

5. **Factors Affecting Release**
   Inhibitors—Hypothalamus (PIH factor), CNS, progesterone
   Stimulators—CNS, suckling stimulus, oxytocin, tranquilizers, PRH (in
        birds)

6. **Deficiency Symptoms**
   Lactation not maintained
   Growth inhibited (some species)

7. **Effects of Overdose, Excess**
   Corpus luteum maintained past normal regression time
   Precocious lactation

METABOLIC ROLE

1. **Biosynthesis**
   Precursors—Amino acids, 20 standard
   Intermediates—Unknown
   Site(s) in cell—Not reported

2. **Production Sites**
   Anterior pituitary—acidophils, E cells
   Placenta

3. **Storage Areas:**   Pituitary

4. **Blood Carriers:**   Free and combined with blood proteins

5. **Half-life:**   Unknown

6. **Target Tissues:**   Mammary gland, ovary, crop sac (pigeons)

7. **Reactions**
   Reactive form—Unknown
   Enzyme systems—Unknown

8. Mode of Action
    Cellular
         Anabolic—Protein synthesis (some species)
         Catabolic—Unknown
         Other—Unknown
    Organismal
         Initiates and maintains lactation
         Increases life of corpus luteum
         Increases weight and growth
         Releases progesterone (in mouse and rat)

9. Catabolism
         Intermediates—Unknown
         Excretion Products—Free in urine; also breakdown products

MISCELLANEOUS

1. **Relationship to Vitamins:** None specifically; all indirectly via growth
    action in species where applicable

2. **Relationship to Other Hormones**
         Progesterone, STH, T4, PTH, Estradiol, Cortisol, Oxytocin—Synergists
         with prolactin [STH, prolactin, ACTH (or adrenal steroids) needed
         for lactation in rats]

3. **Unusual Features**
         Not stimulated, but is inhibited, by hypothalamus (PIH) (except in
         birds)
         Only anterior pituitary hormone precipitated with 0.5% TCA
         Present in male pituitary (human) and probably in blood of male
         Human prolactin not separated from HGH
         HGH stimulates pigeon crop, lactogenic activity in rabbits + luteotrophic
         activity in mouse
         New plumage stimulated in birds by prolactin.
         Antigonadal in male bird; otherwise no known functions in male
         Terminal ring similar to oxytocin ring structure
         Different functions in various species

4. **Possible Relationships of Deficiency Symptoms to Metabolic Action**
         Lactation not maintained—Metabolic functions of prolactin absent
         Growth inhibited—Prolactin needed to synergise growth hormone in
         certain species

22
Adrenocortico-
tropic Hormone
(ACTH)

GENERAL INFORMATION

1. **Synonyms:** Adrenocorticotrop(h)in, corticotrop(h)ic hormone, adreno-corticotrop(h)ic hormone

2. **History**
   - 1930—Smith, P. E., first observed direct relationship between the pituitary and the adrenal cortex
   - 1933—Collip *et al.*; Evans; Houssay *et al.* noted that cell-free extracts of anterior pituitary stimulate adrenal cortex of hypophysectomized animal
   - 1943—Li *et al.*; Sayers *et al.* isolated from anterior pituitary, protein hormones that stimulate adrenal cortex
   - 1954—Bell analyzed amino acid sequence of ACTH
   - 1961—Hofmann ⎫
   - 1963—Li   ⎬ Synthesized ACTH

3. **Physiological Forms:** A_2 (high MW); A_1 (low MW)

4. **Active Analogs and Related Compounds**
   - ACTH sequence 1-21 (100% active)
   - ACTH sequence 1-20 (30% active)
   - ACTH sequence 1-19 with substitutions on #1, 11, 18 (>100% active as ACTH)
   - β-Lipotropin (sheep, pig, beef)

5. **Inactive Analogs and Related Compounds:** α-MSH, β-MSH, ACTH sequence 2-39

6. **Antagonists:** Insulin; concentration dependent for corticosterone, cortisol; STH (protein metabolism)

7. **Synergists:** Epinephrine, cortisol, corticosterone, STH (fat metabolism)

8. **Physiological Functions**
   Maintenance of adrenal cortex
   Promotes secretion of steroids, oxidative phosphorylation in adrenal cortex
   Mobilizes and increases oxidation of free fatty acids in adipose tissue
   Increases gluconeogenesis in liver; increases cyclic AMP in adrenal cortex
   Decreases urea formation in liver

9. **Deficiency Diseases, Disorders:** Adrenal insufficiency; hypopituitarism; Addison's disease (deficiency); Cushing's syndrome (excess); Simmonds' disease (deficiency)

10. **Essentiality for Life**
   One of the most essential hormones—absence causes notable shortening of normal life span

CHEMISTRY

1. **Structure**
   Straight chain, simple polypeptide, 39 amino acids, $C_{214}H_{386}O_{93}N_{56}S$. Structure known and synthesized. Human ACTH: Ser—Tyr—Ser—Met—Glu—His—Phe—Arg—Try—Gly—Lys—Pro—Val—Gly—Lys—Lys—Arg—Arg—Pro—Val—Lys—Val—Tyr—Pro—Asp—Ala—Gly—Glu—Asp—Glu—Ser—Ala—Glu—Ala—Phe—Pro—Leu—Glu—Phe
   No S—S bridges
   Amino acids #1-24 essential, same in all species

2. **Reactions**

Heat—Stable	Alkali
Acid	Inactivates
Weak—stable	Hydrolysis
Strong—hydrolysis	Water—Soluble, acidic

Oxidation

    Irreversibly inactivates using periodate

    Reversibly inactivates using H_2O_2

Reduction—Stable

Light—Stable

Proteolysis—50% digestion of C-terminal end leaves active core

3. Properties

Appearance—White powder

MW—4500 (39 amino acids)

MP—No data

Crystal Form—No data

Salts—No data

Important Groups for Activity

    Methionine—redox center— reacts with thiol; if change proline at #12, 19, 24 or serine #1, lose activity; 1-24 essential

Solubility

    H_2O—Freely sol.

    Acet., Alc.—Sol. in 60% alc., 60% Acet.

    Benz., Chl., Eth.—Insol.

Absn. Max.—Approx. 280 mμ

Chemical Nature—Acidic polypeptide

Misc.—pI = 4.65-4.80

4. Commercial Production

Extract pig, cattle, sheep, whale pituitaries

Synthetic production possible

5. Isolation

Sources—Pituitaries of various animals

Method

Extract with 1 N acetic acid; precipitate with ethanol

Adsorb on and elute from oxycellulose; freeze-dry

Countercurrent distribution—500X purification using s-butanol—0.2% TCA

Zone electrophoresis, end group analysis, analytical ultracentrifugation

6. Determination

Bioassay

Maintenance of weight of adrenal gland in hypophysectomized rats

Depletion of vit. C in adrenals of hypophysectomized rats

Involution of thymus

Physicochemical

Immunoassay

Radioimmunoassay

MEDICAL AND BIOLOGICAL ROLE

1. **Species Occurrence, Specificity, Antigenicity**
   Occurrence—All vertebrates
   Specificity—Slight biological differences, species differences located in
      sequence of amino acids 25-34
   Antigenicity—Slight

2. **Units:**   1 USP unit = 1 I.U. = 1.14 mg

3. **Normal Blood Levels (Man):**   0.0005 unit/100 ml

4. **Administration**
   Injection—Intravenous, intramuscular, subcutaneous
   Topical—No data
   Oral—Active (stimulates release of cortisol)

5. **Factors Affecting Release**
   Inhibitors—Increased plasma level glucocorticoids (feedback)
   Stimulators
      Cortical release factors (CRH)—diurnal rhythm
      Vasopressin, increased hepatic inactivation
      Epinephrine, histamine
      Stimulation of median eminence
      Psychic trauma (via hypothalamus)
      Decreased level of glucocorticoids

6. **Deficiency Symptoms**
   Decreased weight of adrenal (atrophy)
   Decreased mobilization of free fatty acids
   Decreased steroids in blood, urine (17-hydroxy and 17-keto)
   Fasting hypoglycemia
   Increased insulin sensitivity

7. **Effects of Overdose, Excess**
   Increased cortical secretions → hypertrophy → destruction
   Increased pigmentation
   Death
   Hypersensitivity

METABOLIC ROLE

1. **Biosynthesis**
   Precursors—16 of 20 standard amino acids. No Cys, Thr, Ile or Asn
   Intermediates—MSH (?)

2. **Production Sites:** Anterior pituitary—basophilic cells; placenta

3. **Storage Areas:** Anterior pituitary

4. **Blood Carriers:** Free and combined with plasma proteins

5. **Half-life:** 15 min

6. **Target Tissues:** Adrenal cortex, perirenal cells, embryonic rest cells

7. **Reactions**
   Reactive intermediate: cyclic AMP—Secondary messenger

Organ	Enzyme System	Effect
Adrenal cortex	Adenyl cyclase	Activated
	Phosphorylase b	Activated
	Cholesterol 20-Hydroxylase	Activated

8. **Mode of Action**
   Cellular—
   Anabolic—
   Increases melanin synthesis in skin
   Increases steroid synthesis in adrenal
   Increases protein synthesis in liver (via cortisol)
   Catabolic
   Increases glycogenolysis (adrenal cortex)
   Increases gluconeogenesis (liver) (via cortisol)
   Increases lipolysis and oxidation of fatty acids in adipose tissue
   Other:
   Increases oxidative phosphorylation in adrenal cortex
   Increases production of cyclic AMP to produce $NADPH_2$ in adrenal
   cortex
   Decreases cholesterol in adrenal cortex
   Organismal
   Increases weight of adrenals, depletes cortex of vit. C.
   Mobilizes free fatty acids from adipose tissue

Hypoglycemic, reduces urea formation
Increases iodine uptake by thyroid
Stimulates secretion of gluco- and mineralocorticoids by adrenal cortex
Stimulates melanophores, darkening of skin

9. Catabolism
Intermediates—Liver destruction
Excretion Products—Free in urine (very little)

MISCELLANEOUS

1. Relationship to Vitamins
Vitamin C—Depleted in adrenal cortex on stimulation by ACTH
Niacin—Production of $NADPH_2$ by ACTH via cyclic AMP
Vitamin D—Antagonized indirectly by ACTH via cortisol action
Biotin and Vitamin A—Adrenocortical insufficiency noted in biotin and vitamin A deficiency
Pantothenic acid, niacin—Synergistic with ACTH in steroid hormone synthesis

2. Relationship to Other Hormones
Epinephrine—Synergist, stimulates release of ACTH.
Cortisol, corticosterone—Synergists or antagonists depending on concentration. Production stimulated by ACTH
CRH—Stimulates release of ACTH
Vasopressin—Similar to CRH, in action
T4 and TSH—ACTH stimulates iodine uptake by thyroid
MSH—MSH is a part of ACTH molecule
Insulin—Antagonist to ACTH
STH—Antagonist (protein metab.) synergist (fat metab.)

3. Unusual Features
Reversible loss of activity on oxidation with H_2O_2
Reacts with thiols
Irreversible deactivation by periodate
First 13 amino acids essential for corticotropic activity
Full activity at first 20 amino acids
MSH, a part of ACTH, and its activity increased by N-acetylation
Second messenger (cyclic AMP) involved in adrenal cortex

4. **Possible Relationships of Deficiency to Metabolic Action**

Atrophy of adrenal cortex—Lack of stimulus from ACTH

Decreased mobilization of fatty acids—Decreased glucocorticoids, increased insulin activity

Decreased steroids in blood and urine—Decreased production of adrenal corticoids

Fasting hypoglycemia—Decreased gluconeogenesis

Increased insulin sensitivity—Insulin antagonism to ACTH and cortisol

23
Melanocyte-Stimulating Hormone (MSH)

GENERAL INFORMATION

1. **Synonyms:** Melanophore (affecting) hormone, melanophore-stimulating hormone, melanotrophin, melanotrophic hormone, chromatophoro-tropic hormone, melanosome-dispersing hormone, pigmentation hormone, β-hormone

2. **History**

   1932—Zondek and Krohn noted factor in intermediate lobe mediating pigmentary responses in lower vertebrates

   1954—Lerner proposed term melanocyte-stimulating hormone for above factor

   1956—Geschwind *et al.* isolated β-MSH from pig pituitary

   1957—Harris and Lerner isolated α-MSH from pig pituitary tissue

   1959—Harris and Roos isolated β-MSH from bovine pituitary

   1960—Dixon isolated β-MSH from human pituitary

   1960—Hofmann *et al.* synthesized derivatives of β-MSH

   1960—Li, Dixon isolated α-MSH from horse pituitary

   1960—Lee *et al.* determined structure of α-MSH

   1963—Schwyzer *et al.* synthesized α-MSH and β-MSH

3. **Physiological Forms**

   I-α-MSH, I-β-MSH (intermedin) (approx equal biological activity)

4. **Active Analogs and Related Compounds**
    Acetylated *N*-terminal (β-MSH and ACTH)
    Common heptapeptide (Met—Glu—His—Phe—Arg—Try—Gly) of α,β-MSH
    and ACTH

5. **Inactive Analogs and Related Compounds**
    ACTH (1% of MSH activity)
    Hydrolyzed fragments of MSH

6. **Antagonists:**   Cortisone, d-amino acid analogs (competitive inhibitors),
    melatonin

7. **Synergists:**   STH, TSH (amphibia), caffeine, theophylline

8. **Physiological Functions**
    Function in mammals is obscure (protection from sunlight?), small effect
    on skin pigmentation
    Expands or contracts pigments in various chromatophores
    Expands melanophore pigments with color changes in amphibia (adapta-
    tion to environment); weak ACTH activity; adipokinetic effect,
    stimulates T4 secretion
    Increases sensitivity to light, decreases dark adaptation time (lower
    vertebrates)

9. **Deficiency Diseases, Disorders**
    Excess—Addison's disease, adrenal insufficiency (darkening)
    Deficiency—Hypopituitarism (light)

10. **Essentiality for Life:**   Not required; present in all vertebrates with
    differing functions

CHEMISTRY

1. **Structure**
    Polypeptide—purified, synthesized, α and β-forms, straight chains
    α, 13 amino acids—Ser—Tyr—Ser—[Met—Glu—His—Phe—Arg—Try—
    Gly]—Lys—Pro—Val
    N-terminal = CH_3CO—, C-terminal = $—NH_2$ similar all species
    β18 amino acids in all species except 22 in human—Ala—Glu—Lys—
    Lys—Asp—Glu—Gly—Pro—Tyr—Arg—Met—Glu—His—Phe—Arg—
    Try—Gly—Ser—Pro—Pro—Lys—Asp
    No S—S bridges

2. Reactions

Heat—Stable
Acid—Stable
Alkali—Stable (potentiates)
Water—Sol., basic

Oxidation—H_2O_2 reversibly
   inactivates
Reduction—thiols reversibly
   inactivate
Light—No effect
Proteolysis—Decreases activity

3. Properties

Appearance—White powder
MW—α 1500 (13 A.A.)
     β 2100-2600 (18-22 A.A.)
Crystal Form—No data
Salts—No data
Important Groups for Activity
   Met (redox center)
   Tyr
   Common hepapeptide in all
     α's, β's, and ACTH
     (Met———Gly)

Solubility
   H_2O—Sol.
   Acet., Alc.—Insol.
   Benz., Chl., Eth.—Insol.
   Absn. Max.—Approx. 280 mμ
Chemical Nature
   Simple, peptides (α—acidic,
     β—basic)
   α-MSH: α_D^{25} = 58.5°C (10% acetic
     acid)
Misc—pI = α 5.5-7.0, β 11.0

4. Commercial Production: Synthetic

5. Isolation

Sources—Human, pig, bovine, pituitary glands, urine, blood
Methods
   β-MSH
   Extract with KCl at pH 5.5; precipitate with salt; adsorb on
      oxycellulose
   Purify via carboxylic acid resin
   Countercurrent distribution (1.2 M urea, 0.2 M ethylenediamine, 0.1
      N HCl)

6. Determination

Bioassay—Darkening of frog skin ($\alpha > \beta$)
Physicochemical
   Photoelectric reflectance assay
   Immunoasay
   Radioimmunoassay

MEDICAL AND BIOLOGICAL ROLE

1. **Species Occurrence, Specificity, and Antigenicity**
   Occurrence: All vertebrates (α-MSH, β-MSH). All preparations similar in
        activity from all animals
   Specificity
        α-MSH—Slight species differences in activity
        β-MSH—Definite species differences in activity
   Antigenicity: α—None. β—Slight

2. **Units:**   Relative to posterior pituitary standard or by weight

3. **Normal Blood Levels (Man):**   0.09 mμg/ml or less

4. **Administration**
   Injection—Subcutaneous
   Topical—Active, used in amphibian experiments
   Oral—Active, used in amphibian experiments

5. **Factors Affecting Release**
   Inhibitors—MIF via hypothalamus, epinephrine, nervous controls, mela-
        tonin
   Stimulators—Metabolic, nervous controls, MRH via hypothalamus

6. **Deficiency Symptoms**
   Lightened skin color (amphibians)
   Chromatophore contraction
   Guanophore expansion

7. **Effects of Overdose, Excess**
   Darkening of skin (amphibians and humans), temporary
   Hyperglycemia

METABOLIC ROLE

1. **Biosynthesis**
   Precursors—13-14 of 20 standard amino acids. Missing (Cys, Asn, Gln,
        Leu, Ile, Thr, Val)
   Intermediates—Unknown

2. **Production Sites**
   Intermediate lobe of pituitary, except in birds, whales, elephants,
        armadillos, where it is in anterior lobe
   Also in posterior lobes

3. **Storage Areas:**   In intermediate lobe of pituitary

4. **Blood Carriers:**   Free and combined with plasma proteins

5. **Half-life:**   1—2 hrs.

6. **Target Tissues:**   Skin (melanophores) (amphibia)

7. **Reactions**
   Reactive intermediates: Cyclic AMP (secondary messenger)

Organ	Enzyme System	Effect
Skin	Adenyl cyclase	Activated
	Tyrosinase, see ACTH enzymes	Activated

8. **Mode of Action**
   Cellular
       Anabolic—Melanin formation
       Catabolic—Blocks glycolytic pathways
       Other—Increases permeability to Na^+, changes protoplasmic viscosity.
         Expands pigments in melanophores
   Organismal
       ACTH function (weak)
       Blocks action of melatonin
       Regulates skin color changes, light adaptations

9. **Catabolism**
       Intermediates—Unknown
       Excretion products—Free in urine; also breakdown products

MISCELLANEOUS

1. **Relationship to Vitamins**
       Vitamin C—Adrenal cortex depleted on ACTH and MSH activity
       Vitamin A—MSH decreases dark adaptation time

2. **Relationship to Other Hormones**
       STH, TSH—Synergists to MSH
       T4—Secretion stimulated by MSH
       Cortisone, melatonin—Antagonist to MSH
       Epinephrine—Inhibitor of MSH release

3. Unusual Features
Very resistant to degradation or inactivation
Reversibly inactivated by oxidation (H_2O_2)
Reduced with thiols
Heptapeptide 4-10 similar to ACTH
α and β forms with similar activity but different a.a. contents

4. Possible Relationships of Deficiency to Metabolic Action
Lightened skin color (amphibia)—No MSH available to promote melanin
dispersion

24
Oxytocin

GENERAL INFORMATION

1. **Synonyms:** Oxytocic hormone, postlobin-O, posterior-lobe principle, Pitocin, lactogogin, uteracon, α-hypophamine

2. **History**

   1906—Dale noted effect of posterior pituitary factor in stimulating uterine contraction

   1928—Kamin *et al.* separated two active fractions from neural lobe: one was active in raising blood pressure in mammals; the other promoted uterine contractions

   1952—Pierce *et al.* isolated oxytocin

   1953—du Vigneaud *et al.* synthesized oxytocin

   1965—Flouret *et al.* synthesized d-oxytocin

3. **Physiological Forms:** l-oxytocin

4. **Active Analogs and Related Compounds**

   Vasopressin

   Isotocin (some fishes)

   8-Isoleucine oxytocin (other fishes, amphibia)

   Arginine vasotocin (all vertebrates, except mammals)

5. **Inactive Analogs and Related Compounds**

   Reduced form of oxytocin, enlarged or smaller ring forms, forms with side chains removed

6. **Antagonists:**   2'-o-methyltyrosine oxytocin

7. **Synergists**
    Uterus—Prolactin, relaxin, estradiol
    Mammary gland—STH, progesterone, estradiol, T4, cortisol

8. **Physiological Functions**
    Uterine contraction, milk ejection, facilitates sperm ascent in female
        tract
    Decreases: Membrane potential of myometrium; BMR, liver glycogen
    Stimulates oviposition in hen, releases LH
    Increases: Blood sugar, urinary Na and K

9. **Deficiency Diseases, Disorders**
    Insufficiency of labor, atonic uterine bleeding

10. **Essentiality for Life:**   Not essential

CHEMISTRY

1. **Structure:**
    Octapeptide—synthesized
    $\overline{Cys-Tyr-Ile-Gln-Asn-Cys}$—Pro—Leu—Gly—$(NH_2)$
    Oxytocin—$C_{43}H_{66}N_{12}O_{12}S_2$

2. **Reactions**

Heat—No data	Oxidation—Stable
Acid—Stable, (weak), unstable (strong)	Reduction—Inactivates (ring opens)
Alkali—Unstable	Light—No data
Water—Sol., basic	Proteolysis by chymotripsin, trypsin or tyrosinase inactivates

3. **Properties**

Appearance—Amorphous white powder	Solubility
MW—1007	H_2O—Soluble
MP—No data	Acet., Alc.—Sl. Sol., Sol.
Crystal Form—No data	Benz., Chl., Ether—Insol.
Salts—Citrate, flavianate	Absn. Max.—Approx. 280 mμ
Important Groups for Activity	Chemical Nature—Basic octapeptide
Ile, Glu, Asp, Leu, Gly, Cys	$\alpha_D^{22} = -26.2°$
Ring (opening inactivates)	Misc.—pI = 7.7

4. **Commercial Production**
    Synthetic, from amino acids
    Posterior pituitary lobe of cattle, sheep (extraction)

5. **Isolation**
    Sources—Posterior lobe of pituitary, cattle
    Methods
        Dissociate from protein with acid hydrolysis
        Electrodialysis, precipitation
        DEAE cellulose, pH 5.5

6. **Determination**
    Bioassay
        Blood pressure drop in chick
        Milk ejection in rat
        Contraction of isolated, uterus of virgin guinea pig
    Physicochemical—No information

MEDICAL AND BIOLOGICAL ROLE

1. **Species Occurrence, Specificity, and Antigenicity**
    Occurrence: Found in most vertebrates, in slightly different forms
    Specificity: Interspecies reactivity—Decrease in action in lower forms
    Antigenicity: Low

2. **Units:**   1 USP unit = approx. 2 μg of pure hormone

3. **Normal Blood Levels (Man):**   0.15-1.5 milliunits/100 ml plasma

4. **Administration**
    Injection—intramuscular, subcutaneous, I.V. drip
    Topical—Nasal spray
    Oral—Inactivated by chymotrypsin in intestine

5. **Factors Affecting Release**
    Inhibitors: No data
    Stimulants: Reflex arcs—Chemical and neural reflexes from suckling,
        milking, from cervix, vagina (dilatation of birth canal); psychic
        events; relaxin

6. **Deficiency Symptoms**
    Delayed uterine contraction in pregnancy
    Decreased milk flow

7. **Effects of Overdose, Excess**
    Tetanic contraction of pregnant uterus
    Increase in milk flow

METABOLIC ROLE

1. **Biosynthesis**
    Precursors—8 of 20 std amino acids. Missing are Glu, Asp, Met, Arg, Lys,
       His, Pro, Try, Phe, Ala, Thr, Ser
    Intermediates: Neurophysin—Peptide complex

2. **Production Sites:**   Hypothalamus (paraventricular nuclei?)

3. **Storage Areas:**   Posterior pituitary and hypothalamus

4. **Blood Carriers:**   Unbound and in loose association with plasma proteins

5. **Half-life:**   9 min in pregnant woman

6. **Target Tissues:**   Uterus (pregnant), mammary gland, other smooth muscle

7. **Reactions:**   Reactive form—No data

8. **Mode of Action**
    Cellular
       Anabolic—No data
       Catabolic—No data
       Other—Contraction of myoepithelial cells around mammary alveoli.
          Contraction of uterine smooth muscle
    Organismal
       Uterine contraction
       Milk ejection
       Vasodilator   ⎱
       Antidiuretic ⎰ in large doses only

9. Catabolism
   Intermediates
      In pregnancy, plasma oxytocinase inactivates
      Oxytocinase formed in placenta breaks down oxytocin
      Removed from plasma by liver, *kidney*, and mammary gland
   Excretion products: A little, free in urine

MISCELLANEOUS

1. **Relationship to Vitamins:**   No data

2. **Relationship to Hormones**
   Vasopressin
      Structurally similar to vasopressin
      Always secreted with vasopressin irrespective of stimulus
   Prolactin—Oxytocin may stimulate release of prolactin
   STH, TSH, ACTH, LH, FSH, Prol.—Anterior pituitary hormones; related
      in milk production
   Estradiol—Uterine effect dependent on estrogen presence.
   LH—oxytocin stimulates LH release
   Norepinephrine ⎫
   Serotonin   ⎬ Occur with oxytocin in posterior pituitary
   CRH—Structural similarity to oxytocin
   Relaxin—Stimulates oxytocin release

3. **Unusual Features**
   Very similar structurally to vasopressin but main physiological actions
      very different (only two amino acids differ)
   No known function in male mammal
   Protein, neurophysin, binds neurohypophysial hormones specifically
   Always secreted with vasopressin irrespective of nature of stimulus
   Nonpregnant uterus is more sensitive to ADH than to oxytocin
   Vasodilator effect of oxytocin is blocked by ADH
   Releases anterior pituitary hormones in fish
   Increases oviposition in birds and reptiles
   Increases spawning reflex in fish

4. **Possible Relationships of Deficiency Symptoms to Metabolic Action:**   No
      data

25
Vasopressin

GENERAL INFORMATION

1. **Synonyms:** Arginine vasopressin, ADH (antidiuretic hormone) antidiuretin, Pitressin, β-hypophamine, Tonephin, Vasophysin

2. **History**
   1895—Oliver and Schafer noted effect of posterior pituitary factor on rise in blood pressure
   1937—Gilman and Goodman showed dehydration increased plasma and urine levels of vasopressin
   1942—Van Dyke isolated crude protein fraction possessing oxytocin and vasopressin activities from oxen pituitaries
   1953-54—DuVigneaud *et al.* determined structure and synthesized ADH

3. **Physiological Forms:** l-vasopressin

4. **Active Analogs and Related Compounds**
   Arginine vasopressin (most mammals)
   Lysine vasopressin (pig)
   Vasotocin (birds, amphibia, fish)

5. **Inactive Analogs and Related Compounds**
   Opening of ring; removal of side chain
   Change in size of ring

6. **Antagonists:** Norepinephrine, certain prostaglandins

7. **Synergists:**   Aldosterone, STH, prolactin, corticosterone, T4, testosterone, epinephrine

8. **Physiological Functions**
    Elevates blood pressure (mammals) (reverse effect in birds)
    Decreases kidney blood flow
    Antidiuretic, acts as CRF, releases ACTH
    Increases NaCl and urea excretion
    Regulates water balance
    Stimulates contraction of smooth muscles
    Increases renal tubular H_2O reabsorption
    Releases anterior pituitary hormones

9. **Deficiency Diseases, Disorders**
    Deficiency—Diabetes insipidus
    Excess—Schwartz-Bartter syndrome (oat-cell carcinoma)

10. **Essentiality for Life:**   Not essential

CHEMISTRY

1. **Structure**
    Octapeptide—synthesized
    Cys—Tyr—Phe—Gln—Asn—Cys—Pro—Arg—Gly(NH$_2$)
    Arginine vasopressin, $C_{46}H_{65}N_{15}O_{12}S_2$

2. **Reactions**

Heat—Degrades in solution	Oxidation—Stable
Acid—Stable	Reduction—Inactivates (ring opens)
Alkali—Unstable	Light—Unstable
Water—Soluble, basic	Proteolysis inactivates (by trypsin (which removes terminal glycine amide group), but not by pepsin)

3. **Properties**

Appearance—amorphous white powder	Important Groups for Activity
MW—1084 (arginine-vasopressin)	Cyclic pentapeptide (opening inactivates)
MP—No data	Tripeptide side chain
Crystal Form—No data	Cys
Salts, Esters—Tannate	

Solubility

    H_2O—Soluble

    Alc.—Sol.

    Acet., Benz., Chl., Eth.—Insol.

Absn. Max.—Approx. 280 mμ

Chemical Nature—Basic peptide

Misc.—pI = 10.9

4. Commercial Production

Synthesized from amino acids.

Posterior lobe of pituitary of domestic animals (hog, beef)

5. Isolation

Sources: Posterior pituitary glands (hog, beef)

Methods:

Acetic acid extraction of posterior pituitary powder

Percolation through Celite using 70% ethanol and gradually increasing concentrations of water and acetic acid

Or the neurophysin peptide complex is extracted with acetic acid and the protein precipitated with NaCl. Treatment with trichloroacetic acid then dissociates the complex and precipitates the protein

6. Determination

Bioassay

Blood pressure measurements on cats, dogs, or chickens

Diuretic studies on dogs, rats, and rabbits

Weight gain in frogs

Physiochemical: Radioimmunoassay

MEDICAL AND BIOLOGICAL ROLE

1. Species Occurrence, Specificity, and Antigenicity

Occurrence

Vasopressin-like substances found in vertebrates from cyclostomes through mammals

Loss of activity as go to amphibia and fish

Specificity—Decreasing interspecies reactivity in lower vertebrates

Antigenicity—Low

2. Units:

1 USP posterior pituitary unit = 1 international posterior pituitary unit = 0.5 mg of the international standard oxytocic, vasopressor, and antidiuretic substances (ox posterior pituitary)

3. Normal Blood Levels (Man):

3.7 milliunits/100 ml

4. **Administration**
    Injection—Intravenous, intramuscular, or subcutaneous
    Topical—Inhalation of powders or sprays
    Oral—No data

5. **Factors Affecting Release**
    Inhibitors
        Low osmotic pressure in blood
        Ethyl alcohol
        High extracellular fluid volume
    Stimulators
        High blood osmotic pressure
        Acetylcholine, lobeline
        Physostigmine
        Cold, low fluid volume
        Hemorrhage
        Morphine, nicotine, ether, some barbiturates, tranquilizers, and
            general anesthetics
        Ca^{++}-ion-(inhibits binding to protein)
        Stress
        Exercise, psychic events

6. **Deficiency Symptoms**
    Diuresis
    Polydipsia
    Decreased NaCl and urea excretion

7. **Effects of Overdose, Excess**
    Increased water reabsorption, blood pressure
    Smooth muscle contraction—G.I. activity
    Facial pallor
    Uterine cramps
    Coronary circulation complications

METABOLIC ROLE

1. **Biosynthesis**
    Precursors—Eight of standard 20 amino acids. Missing are Glu, Asp, Met,
        Lys, His, Leu, Prol, Try, Ile, Ala, Thre, Ser
    Intermediates—Neurophysin-peptide complex

2. **Production Sites:**   Hypothalamus, esp. supraoptic nuclei. Secreted into neurohypophysis

3. **Storage Areas:**   Hypothalamus and posterior pituitary

4. **Blood Carriers:**   Unbound, and loose association with plasma protein

5. **Half-life:**   In plasma, 8 min

6. **Target Tissues:**   Capillaries, arterioles, coronary vessels, kidney tubules, smooth muscle

7. **Reactions**

    Reactive intermediate: Cyclic AMP—secondary messenger

Organ	Enzyme System	Effect
Kidney	Hyaluronidase	Activated
Kidney (distal tubule)	Adenyl cyclase	Activated

8. **Mode of Action**

    Cellular

    Anabolic—No data

    Catabolic—Depolymerizes hyaluronic acid

    Other

    Increases passive permeability of epithelium of distal segment of nephron to water; allows osmotic forces to operate more freely

    Increases intracellular water in muscle; decreases Na and K

    Increases pore size or number in cell membrane

    Organismal

    Antidiuretic

    Decreases coronary blood flow

    Increases motility of bowel

    Arterial smooth muscle sensitized to effects of norepinephrine by physiological amounts of ADH

    Renal blood flow reduced by ADH

9. **Catabolism**

    Intermediates—Inactivated in kidney and liver

    Excretion Products: Some free in urine

MISCELLANEOUS

1. **Relationship to Vitamins:**   No data

2. **Relationship to Other Hormones**

   Oxytocin, Hypertensin—Structurally very similar to vasopressin but main physiological effect is very different

   Aldosterone, Corticosterone—Synergistic with vasopressin; related to antidiuretic activity of vasopressin

   CRF—Vasopressin suggested to have CRF (corticotropin release factor) properties

   STH, T4, Testosterone, Prolactin—Synergistic with vasopressin

   Aldosterone—ADH and aldosterone may interact in water and electrolyte conservation

   Norepinephrine, Prostaglandins—Norepinephrine and certain prostaglandins inhibit ADH activity in kidney

3. **Unusual Features**

   Thiazides which act as diuretics, paradoxically reduce polyuria in both pituitary diabetes insipidus and nephrogenic diabetes insipidus. May act by reducing filtration rate

   Nonpregnant uterus is more sensitive to ADH than to oxytocin. Rare form of diabetes insipidus is not caused by lack of ADH but by inability of kidney tubule to respond to ADH. (An inborn error of metabolism)

   Reverse effects in birds

   Increases skin permeability in amphibia

4. **Possible Relationships of Deficiency Symptoms to Metabolic Action**

   Decreased NaCl and urea excretion—Permeability of epithelium of distal segment of nephron to water is reduced and water reabsorption is decreased

26
Thyroxine

GENERAL INFORMATION

1. **Synonyms:** T_4, 3,5,3',5'-tetraiodothyronine

2. **History**

   16th Century—Anon. Cretinism described

   1825—Parry associated enlarged thyroid with exophthalmia, tachycardia

   1874—Gull associated atrophy of thyroid with characteristic syndrome

   1891—Murray treated hypothyroidism with injection of thyroid extract

   1896—Baumann showed that thyroid contains iodine

   1911—Baumann demonstrated diiodotyrosine in thyroid

   1915—Kendall isolated and crystallized thyroxine

   1926—Harington determined structural formula

   1927—Harington and Barger synthesized thyroxine

   1951—Gross *et al.* isolated and identified triiodothyronine as active factor in thyroid

3. **Physiological Forms:** l-thyroxine, 3',3,5-triiodothyronine (T_3, TRIT), tetraiodothyroacetic acid (TETRAC), triiodothyroacetic acid (TRIAC)

4. **Active Analogs and Related Compounds**

   d-thyroxine (fractional activity of l-thyroxine)

   Triiodothyropropionic acid (very active in tadpole metamorphosis)

5. **Inactive Analogs and Related Compounds:** Deiodinated T4; T4 with esterified hydroxyl group

6. **Antagonists:**   3,3',5'-triiodothyronine, guanethidine; 2',6'-diiodotyrosine, insulin, PTH

7. **Synergists:**   STH, cortisol, epinephrine, prolactin, MSH, oxytocin, progesterone, vasopressin

8. **Physiological Functions**
    Regulates growth, differentiation, oxidative metabolism, electrolytic balance
    Increases CHO metabolism, calorigenesis, protein anabolism, BMR, O_2 consumption, fat catabolism, fertility
    Sensitizes nervous system

9. **Deficiency Diseases, Disorders**
    Deficiency—Cretinism, goiter (deficient), Hashimoto's disease, Gull's disease, myxedema
    Excess—Grave's disease, thyrotoxicosis, thyroiditis, goiter

10. **Essentiality for Life**
    Required for development and growth of all vertebrates
    Deficiency in adult shortens life span

CHEMISTRY

1. **Structure:**

Thyroxine, $C_{15}H_{11}I_4NO_4$

2. **Reactions**

Heat—Decomposes at 231°C	Oxidation—Unstable
Acid—Unstable (Sol. in acid alc.)	Reduction—Stable
	Light—Unstable
Alkali—Sol. in alk. alc.	Enzyme action: Unstable to
Water—Insol.	deiodinating enzymes.

3. **Properties**

Appearance—White crystalline powder

MW—776.9

MP—231-233°C decomp.

Crystal Form—needle-like

Salts—Sodium

Important Groups for Activity

—l-Alanine

—O—

—I (all 4 positions)

—OH

Solubility

H_2O—Insol.

Acet.—Insol.

Alc.—Sol. at acid or alk. pH

Benz., Chl., Eth.—Insol.

Absn. Max.—231 mμ

Chemical Nature

Acidic substituted amino acid

α_D = −4.4° (aq. alk. EtOH)

Misc.—pK_a = 2.2, (COOH), 6.45 (OH), 10.1 (NH_2)

pI = 3.5

4. **Commercial Production**

Synthetic and from pig thyroid by defatting and drying with acetone— thyroid, U.S.P.

Sodium salts

Sodium levothyroxine, USP (synthroid)

Sodium liothyronine, USP (cytomel)

5. **Isolation**

Sources—Pig thyroid

Method—Extraction:

Proteolysis, pH 8.4, (pancreatin and trypsin) of thyroid, 24 hr at 37°C

Extract with *n*-butanol saturated with *N* HCl

Paper chromatography or ion-exchange resin

Partition chromatography (kieselguhr in 0.5 *N* NaOH) separates T_4 from T_3

6. **Determination**

Bioassay

Metamorphosis in tadpoles

Increased oxidative metabolism

Physicochemical—Protein-bound iodine (PBI) in plasma. Radioassay

MEDICAL AND BIOLOGICAL ROLE

1. **Species Occurrence, Specificity, and Antigenicity**
    Occurrence
    　　All vertebrates have thyroid tissue, but follicles dispersed in lampreys
    　　　and bony fish
    　　Thyroxine and precursors found in various invertebrates but no
    　　　follicles
    Specificity
    　　Interreactive all vertebrates; no loss in potency (i.e. no specificity)
    　　No response in invertebrates; different functions in lower vertebrates
    Antigenicity—No antigenicity

2. **Units:** In mg

3. **Normal Blood Levels (Man):** 3.0-6.5 μg/100 ml serum

4. **Administration:**
    Injection—No data
    Topical—No data
    Oral—Thyroid tablets, sodium levothyroxine, sodium liothyroxine

5. **Factors Affecting Release**
    Inhibitors
    　　High blood I_2
    　　High blood T_4—feedback via hypothalamus
    　　Stress, pain
    Stimulators
    　　TSH
    　　Low blood T_4—feedback via hypothalamus
    　　Cold
    　　Direct nervous control

6. **Deficiency Symptoms (Humans)**
    Tumors of pituitary
    Decreased BMR
    Accumulation of mucoprotein
    Increase in blood lipid and cholesterol
    Increase in liver gluconeogenesis
    Extracellular retention of NaCl and H_2O

7. **Effects of Overdose, Excess**
   Acceleration of growth, maturation
   Increased BMR, esp. liver, skin, kidney, smooth muscle, gastric mucosa
   Decreased tissue glycogen
   Increased blood sugar
   Exophthalmos
   Hyperthyroidism, Graves's disease
   Thyrotoxicosis

METABOLIC ROLE

1. **Biosynthesis:**   Tyrosine → Monoiodotyrosine → Diiodotyrosine → Thyroxine Site(s) in Cell—Data not conclusive

2. **Production Sites:**   Thyroid gland

3. **Storage Areas:**   Colloid in thyroid follicles = thyroglobulin

4. **Blood Carriers**
   α-Globulin
   Acid glycoprotein
   Albumin

5. **Half-life:**   6-7 days

6. **Target Tissues:**   Systemic—All tissues, esp. adenohypophysis, hypothalamus

7. **Reactions**
   Reactive intermediate: Cyclic AMP—secondary messenger

Organ	Enzyme System	Effect
	67 tissue enzymes affected *in vivo*	
Thyroid	Mitochondrial enzyme systems	Activated
Thyroid	TCA cycle—oxidative phosphorylating enzymes	Uncoupled
Thyroid	Adenyl cyclase	Activated

8. **Mode of Action**
   Cellular
   Anabolic
   Increases protein synthesis on the ribosomes and $_m$RNA synthesis in muscle, kidney, reticulocytes, liver

Catabolic
Increases protein catabolism in brain, spleen, and testis
Increases glucose and fat catabolism
Other—Swells mitochondria, affects permeability, regulates redox
potential, chelates metals that inhibit enzymes
Uncouples mitochondrial oxidative phosphorylation at 2 points
Decreases mucoprotein synthesis
Organismal
Stimulates hematopoiesis, oögenesis, spermatogenesis, lactation,
intestinal absorption
Regulates growth, differentiation, electrolyte balance, heat produc-
tion, O_2 consumption, BMR
Sensitizes nervous system

9. **Catabolism**
Intermediates
Iodine split off in liver, kidney, salivary glands, and recycled
Residue coupled with glucuronic acid or sulfate and excreted. Also
oxidative deamination of amino acid residues
Excretion Products
Compounds containing diphenyl ether and at least two carbons of side
chain excreted as glucuronides and sulfates in bile
Very small amounts free in urine and bile

MISCELLANEOUS

1. **Relationship to Vitamins**
Vitamin A—T_4 needed for vit. A synthesis in liver
B—Complex vitamin deficiencies develop in hyperthyroidism
Vit B_{12}—T4 aids in B_{12} absorption
Vitamin C—Synergist in cold survival
Niacin—Synergist in mitochondrial metabolism

2. **Relationship to Other Hormones**
STH, ACTH, FSH, LH, TSH, Prolactin—synergists to T4 esp. in
lactation
ACTH—Antagonist in proper relative concentration
Insulin—T4 stimulates secretion of insulin
TSH—Stimulates production of T4
FSH—Inhibited by T4
MSH, ACTH—Stimulate iodine uptake by thyroid

PTH—Antagonist to T4
Cortisol—Synergist to T4

3. **Unusual Features**
    Powerful chelating agent, esp. with Mg
    Free OH participates in quinonoid formation
    Regulates metamorphosis in amphibia
    Osmoregulatory in fish
    Iodinated tyrosine found in invertebrate exoskeleton—inactive
    Diffuse thyroid gland in teleosts & other lower forms
    TRIAC—potent stimulant for metamorphosis
    TETRAC—potent metabolic stimulant
    Decreased activity if I is replaced with Br or Cl
    Decreased activity if OH is removed or I position changed

4. **Possible Relationships of Deficiency Symptoms to Metabolic Action**
    Decreased BMR—Lack of T_4 stimulus for anabolism
    Accumulation of Mucoprotein—Lack of T_4 control of mucoprotein
        synthesis
    Increase in Blood Lipid and Cholesterol—Decreased fat catabolism
    Increase in Liver Gluconeogenesis—Antagonism by ACTH (cortisol)
    Extracellular Retention of NaCl and H_2O—Antagonism by ACTH and
        aldosterone (?)

27
Parathyroid
Hormone

GENERAL INFORMATION

1. **Synonyms:** PTH, Parathormone

2. **History**
   1900—Vassale and Generali reported convulsions and tetany from removal of parathyroids only
   1909—MacCallum and Voegtlin reported effect of parathyroidectomy on plasma Ca
   1924-25—Hanson, Collip prepared active extracts from parathyroid gland
   1942—Patt and Luckhardt demonstrated that blood Ca level controls parathyroid secretion
   1959—Rasmussen, Aurbach prepared pure parathyroid hormone peptides

3. **Physiological Forms:** /-Parathormone

4. **Active Analogs and Related Compounds:** No data

5. **Inactive Analogs and Related Compounds:** No data

6. **Antagonists:** T4, STH, estradiol, testosterone, TCT

7. **Synergists:** Vitamin D, estrogens (birds), cortisol

8. **Physiological Functions**

Increases blood Ca, kidney Ca reabsorption, PO_4 excretion, blood citrate
Mobilizes Ca and PO_4 from bone.
Activates Ca and PO_4 absorption from G.I. tract (requires vitamin D)
Increases osteoclast formation

9. **Deficiency Diseases, Disorders**

Deficiency—Tetany, hypoparathyroidism
Excess—von Recklinghausen's disease, hyperparathyroidism

10. **Essentiality for Life:**   One of the most essential hormones. Absence
rapidly leads to tetany and death of adult

CHEMISTRY

1. **Structure**

Simple polypeptide (83 amino acids), sequence determined
Straight chain—No S—S bridges
Ala———Leu

2. **Reactions**

Heat—No data
Acid—Stable, dilute, acid
Alkali—Relatively unstable
Water—Sol., acidic

Oxidation—H_2O_2, performic
  acid inactivate
Reduction—Stable
Light—No data
Proteolysis—Loses activity

3. **Properties**

Appearance—No data
MW—8500
MP—No data
Crystal Form—No data
Salts—No data
Important Groups for Activity
  Met, Try, Tyr

Solubility
  H_2O—Sol.
  Acet., Alc.—Insol.
  Benz., Chl., Eth.—Insol.
Absn. Max.—Approx. 280 mμ
Chemical Nature—Acidic
  polypeptide
Misc—pl = 4.8

4. **Commercial Production:**   From bovine parathyroid

5. **Isolation**

Sources—Bovine parathyroid

Methods
    Extraction
        Extract with 80% acetic acid
        Precipitate in 86% acetone
        Ultrafilter at pH 2.4
    Purification
        Column chromatography on Dowex 50
        Countercurrent distribution
        Gel filtration

6. Determination
    Bioassay
        Serum Ca increase in dogs
        Increase in urine P output
    Physicochemical
        Radioimmunoassay

MEDICAL AND BIOLOGICAL ROLE

1. Species Occurrence, Specificity, and Antigenicity
    Occurrence—Found in all vertebrates above fish and cyclostomes
    Specificity—Interspecific potency high, e.g. bovine and human Para-
        thormone—Isoactive
    Antigenicity—Low

2. Units: 1 USP unit = 1/100 the amount of PTH to increase dog blood Ca
    1 mg/100 ml in 18 hr after subcutaneous injection

3. Normal Blood Levels (Man): Est. 4000 USP units/100 ml plasma

4. Administration
    Injection—Parathyroid USP (Paroidin) usually subcutaneous; occasion-
        ally I.V.
    Topical—No data
    Oral—Destroyed by proteolytic enzymes

5. Factors Affecting Release
    Inhibitors—High serum Ca; vasomotor nerve control
    Stimulators—Low serum Ca feedback; vasomotor nerve control

6. **Deficiency Symptoms**
   Decreased blood (Ca, citrate), urine (PO_4, Ca).
   Increased blood PO_4.
   Irritability of nervous system, muscle twitch, tetany, death
   Cataracts

7. **Effects of Overdose, Excess**
   Increased blood (Ca, citrate, alkaline phosphatase), urine PO_4, demineralization of skeleton, osteoclast activity
   Decreased blood PO_4, muscle sensitivity
   Metastatic deposits of Ca in tissues, notably kidney

METABOLIC ROLE

1. **Biosynthesis**
   Precursors—17 of 20 standard amino acids. No Cys, Asn, or Gln
   Intermediates—No data
   Site(s) in cell—No data

2. **Production Sites:**   Parathyroid gland. Principal cells (?)

3. **Storage Areas:**   No data

4. **Blood Carriers:** α-globulin and albumin

5. **Half-life:**   20 min

6. **Target Tissues:**   Bone, kidney, muscle, mammary gland, gut

7. **Reactions:**   Reactive intermediate—Cyclic AMP—secondary messenger

Organ	Enzyme System	Effect
Bone and Kidney	Adenyl cyclase	Activated

8. **Mode of Action**
   Cellular
     Anabolic—No data
     Catabolic—Bone resorption
     Other
       Mitochondrial PO_4 increased

        Mitochondrial swelling
        Increased conversion pyruvate to citrate
    Organismal
        Raises renal Ca threshold
        Lowers renal PO_4 threshold

9. Catabolism
Intermediates—Partial digestion in liver
Excretion Products—1% in urine

MISCELLANEOUS

1. Relationship to Vitamins
Vitamin D—Synergistic with PTH in maintenance of serum calcium

2. Relationship to Other Hormones
Estradiol—Synergises PTH in birds
Cortisol—Synergises PTH in vertebrates
T4, STH, Estradiol, Testosterone, Calcitonin—Antagonists to PTH

3. Unusual Features
Activity increased with molecular weight of analog
Demineralization of skeleton, formation of cysts with excess PTH
High citrate produced in bone action

4. Possible Relationships of Deficiency Symptoms to Metabolic Action
Decreased blood Ca, citrate—Lack of PTH mobilization of bone calcium
Increased blood PO_4—Urine threshold for PO_4 high without PTH
Irritability of nervous system—Decrease of blood calcium
Cataracts—?

28
Thyrocalcitonin

GENERAL INFORMATION

1. **Synonyms:** TCT, calcitonin

2. **History**
   1962—Copp discovered and named hormone with effects opposite to those of Parathormone
   1963—Munson extracted thyrocalcitonin from rat thyroids
   1964—Foster *et al*. reported that calcitonin originated in thyroid gland in goats
   1966—Pearse identified thyroid "C" cells as source of calcitonin

3. **Physiological Forms:** l-Thyrocalcitonin

4. **Active Analogs and Related Compounds:** No data

5. **Inactive Analogs and Related Compounds:** No data

6. **Antagonists:** Parathyroid hormone, vit. D

7. **Synergists:** Estradiol

8. **Physiological Functions**
   Decreases blood Ca [balances PTH (parathyroid hormone)]
   Inhibits bone resorption

Increases PO_4 excretion

Increases proline incorporation into bone

9. **Deficiency Diseases, Disorders:**   Medullary carcinoma of the thyroid (excess)

10. **Essentiality for Life:**   Not demonstrated

CHEMISTRY

1. **Structure**

    Polypeptide, 32 amino acids, synthesized

    Straight chain, one S—S ring: Porcine TCT Cys—Ser—Asn—Leu—Ser—
        Thr—Cys—Val—Leu—Ser—Ala—Try—Trp—Arg—Asn—Leu—Asn—
        Asn—Phe—His—Arg—Phe—Ser—Gly—Met—Gly—Phe—Gly—Pro—
        Glu—Thr—Pro

2. **Reactions**

    Heat—Relatively stable   Oxidation—No data
    Acid—Sol., Inactivates (conc.)   Reduction—No data
    Alkali—Inactivates (conc.)   Light—No data
    Water—Sol., acidic   Proteolysis—Pepsin and
                                                trypsin inactivates

3. **Properties**

    Appearance—No data   Solubility
    MW—3604 H_2O—Sol.
    MP—No data   Acet., Alc.—Insol.
    Crystal Form—No Data   Benz., Chl., Eth.—Insol.
    Salts—No data   Absn. Max.—Approx 280 mμ
    Important Groups for Activity   Chemical Nature—Acidic
        S—S ring 1 + 7 position   polypeptide
        Tyr and Try in   Misc.—pI = 4.8
            positions 12 and 13

4. **Commercial Production:**   Not available

5. **Isolation**

    Sources—Pork thyroid

Method
> Extraction
>> (a) Extract with 0.2 N HCl 60-70°C for 5 min, filter after 1 hr
>> (b) Dialyze, pH 4.6, against 0.1 M acetate buffer at 4°C
>> (c) Precipitate from 1.5 M NaCl
> Purification
>> (a) Gel filtration—Sephadex G-100, pH 4.6
>> (b) Ultrafiltration—If complexed to proteins earlier

6. **Determination**
   Bioassay—Effect on plasma Ca level in rat
   Physicochemical—Radioimmunoassay

MEDICAL AND BIOLOGICAL ROLE

1. **Species Occurrence, Specificity, and Antigenicity**
   Occurrence—Found in most vertebrates
   Specificity—High, great variation in interspecific potency
   Antigenicity—Not antigenic

2. **Units**
   MRC units or by weight
   5-10 MRC milliunits lowers plasma Ca in rat by about 10%

3. **Normal Blood Levels:**   0.01 μg/100 ml plasma (rabbit)

4. **Administration**
   Injection—Active
   Topical—Inactive
   Oral—Inactive

5. **Factors Affecting Release**
   Inhibitors—No data
   Stimulators—High plasma calcium level, glucagon

6. **Deficiency Symptoms:**   Blood Ca increase

7. **Effects of Overdose, Excess:**   Blood Ca decrease

METABOLIC ROLE

1. **Biosynthesis**
   Precursors—18 of 20 standard amino acids; Lys, Ile absent
   Intermediates—Unknown
   Site(s) in cell—Unknown

2. **Production Sites**
   Thyroid, parathyroid, and thymus (man)
   Parafollicular C cells derived from ultimobranchial body

3. **Storage Areas:**   Unknown

4. **Blood Carriers:**   Unknown

5. **Half-life:**   5-15 min (rabbit)

6. **Target Tissues:**   Bone, kidney, muscle

7. **Reactions**
   Reactive intermediate—Cyclic AMP—secondary messenger

Organ	Enzyme System	Effect
Thyroid	Adenyl cyclase	Activated
	Phosphorylase b	Activated

8. **Mode of Action**
   Cellular
       Anabolic—Increases proline incorporation into bone
       Catabolic—No data
       Other—No data
   Organismal
       Decreases blood calcium
       Inhibits bone resorption and citrate formation
       Increases PO_4 excretion
       Decreases glucose utilization and lactate production in bone

9. **Catabolism**
   Intermediates—Liver proteolysis
   Excretion products—Products of protein metabolism

MISCELLANEOUS

1. **Relationship to Vitamins:**   Vitamin D antagonizes TCT

2. **Relationship to Other Hormones**
   PTH—Antagonist to thyrocalcitonin
   Glucagon—Stimulates release of TCT
   Estradiol—Synergises and releases TCT

3. **Unusual Features:**   Birds have a gland separate from thyroid containing
   TCT

4. **Possible Relationships of Deficiency to Metabolic Action**
   Blood calcium increase—Unknown

29
Insulin

GENERAL INFORMATION

1. **Synonyms:**   None

2. **History**

      10 A.D.—Celsus described diabetic syndrome
      1899—Von Mering and Minkowski demonstrated relationship between pancreatectomy and diabetes mellitus
      1922—Macleod determined that islet cells produce insulin
      1922—Banting and Best prepared potent insulin extracts from dog pancreas
      1926—Abel *et al.* isolated crystalline insulin
      1955—Sanger *et al.* determined structure of insulin
      1966—Katsoyannis synthesized insulin (human and sheep)

3. **Physiological Forms:**   l-Insulin

4. **Active Analogs and Related Compounds:**   No data

5. **Inactive Analogs and Related Compounds**
      Oxidized, reduced insulin, proinsulin
      Alkali inactivated insulin

6. **Antagonists:**   Cortisol, glucagon, epinephrine, norepinephrine, STH (CHO and fat metabolism), T4

7. **Synergists:**   STH (protein metabolism), testosterone, estradiol

8. **Physiological Function**
   Regulates CHO and fat metabolism, esp. glucose and fat oxidations
   Stimulates amino acid and glucose transport into cells and protein synthesis
   Stimulates glycogen and mucopolysaccharide formation

9. **Deficiency Diseases, Disorders:**   Diabetes mellitus (faulty β-cells), azoturia, hyperlipemia, ketonemia

10. **Essentiality for Life:**   Essential for survival

CHEMISTRY

1. **Structure**
   Structure known and synthesized—51 amino acids
   Polypeptide, 2 parallel straight chains, -3— S—S bridges
   2 chains (ox insulin)
   α—21 amino acids—acidic: Gly—Ile—Val—Glu—Glu—
   Cys—Cys—Ala—Ser—Val—Cys—Ser—Leu—Tyr—Glu—Leu—Glu—
   Asp—Tyr—Cys—Asp
   β—30 amino acids—basic: Phe—Val—Asp—Glu—His—Leu—Cys—Gly—
   Ser—His—Leu—Val—Glu—Ala—Leu—Tyr—Leu—Val—Cys—Gly—
   Glu—Arg—Gly—Phe—Phe—Tyr—Thr—Pro—Lys—Ala

2. **Reactions**

Heat—Unstable	Oxidation—Inactivates
Acid—Stable	Reduction—Inactivates
Alkali—Inactivates	Light—No data
Water—Soluble, acidic	Proteolysis—Trypsin inactivates

3. **Properties**

Appearance—White crystalline powder	Important Groups for Activity
	2 Disulfide bridges (S—S ring)
MW—5734 monomer	Active groups unknown
Polymer: 12,000-48,000, depending on pH	Key positions—19-21 on α-chain; 22-30 on β-chain
MP—No data	Tyr, Asn
Crystal Form—Hexagonal system	
Salts—Zinc, Protamine	

Solubility	Absn. Max.—Approx. 280 mμ
H_2O—Soluble	Chemical Nature—Acidic
Acet., Alc.—Sol.	polypeptide
Benz., Chl., Eth.—Insol.	Misc.—pI = 5.3

4. Commercial Production: Extraction of beef or pork pancreas

5. Isolation

Sources—Pancreas—beef, pork

Method

Extract pancreas in 80% EtOH, pH 3 (H_3PO_4)

pH to 8 with NH_4OH precipitates impurities

Precipitate insulin with EtOH and ether

Dissolve in EtOH—H_3PO_4 buffer and precipitate insulin as picrate

Dissolve in acetone HCl

Precipitate with acetone

Wash and dry

Purification

Crystallize at pI in acetate buffer with 0.15-0.60% zinc

Precipitate with alc.

Salting out

Gel filtration and crystallization or electrophoresis

6. Determination

Bioassay

Isolated rat diaphragm; perfused heart; *in vitro* systems, for measuring glucose uptake

Lowering blood sugar in rabbit

Physicochemical

Radioimmunoassay

Immunoassay—Very sensitive for plasma insulin concentration

MEDICAL AND BIOLOGICAL ROLE

1. Species Occurrence, Specificity, and Antigenicity

Occurrence—Found in all vertebrates

Specificity—Moderate interspecific potency

Antigenicity—Moderate antigenicity. Pig and human sequence alike yet antigenic differences exist

2. Units: 1 I.U. = 1 USP unit = 0.04167 mg international standard

3. **Normal Blood Levels:** $0.1\text{-}3.0 \times 10^{-3}$ I.U./ml

4. **Administration**
   Injection—Subcutaneous
      Amorphous Insulin, Crystalline Insulin—Fact acting, short duration
      Protamine Insulin, Protamine Zn insulin—Slow, steady absorption
   Topical—Not used
   Oral
      Sulfonylureas—Stimulate secretion of insulin
      Hypoglycemic agents—Stimulate secretion of insulin
      Biguanides—Stimulate secretion of insulin

5. **Factors Affecting Release**
   Inhibitors
      Low blood sugar—Feedback
      Epinephrine
      Norepinephrine
   Stimulators
      High blood sugar—Feedback
      Elevated blood amino acid level
      Vagal stimulation
      Glucagon, ACTH, secretin, STH,
      Ketone bodies, sulfonylureas, biguanides
      Hypoglycemic agents
      Cortisol, T4

6. **Deficiency Symptoms**
   Polyphagia
   Decreases respiratory quotient
   Decreases tissue protein
   Polydipsia
   Hyperglycemia, Glycosuria—Underutilization and overproduction of
      glucose
   Polyurea
   Hyperlipemia
   Ketonemia
   Azoturia

7. **Effects of Overdose, Excess**
   Convulsions
   Increases glycogen storage
   Mental confusion

Coma
Headache
Tremor
Sweating
Apprehensiveness

METABOLIC ROLE

1. **Biosynthesis**
   Precursors—17 of 20 standard amino acids (aspartic acid, tryptophan, and methionine missing)
   Intermediates—Proinsulin
   Site(s) in cell—Unknown

2. **Production Sites:** β-cells of islets of pancreas

3. **Storage Areas:** β-granules in β-cells

4. **Blood Carriers:** Circulating proteins; α,β-macroglobulins

5. **Half-life in Plasma:** Nonlabeled insulin, < 9 min; insulin ^{131}I, 40 min

6. **Target Tissues:** Systemic, esp. liver, adipose tissue, muscle, kidney.

7. **Reactions:** Reactive form—unknown

Organ	Enzyme System	Effect
Liver	Lipase	Inhibited
	Adenyl cyclase	Inhibited
	Glycogen synthetase	Activated
Tissues	Hexokinase	Activated
	Phosphorylases	Activated

8. **Mode of Action**
   Cellular
      Anabolic—Increases mucopolysaccharide synthesis, protein synthesis, fatty acid synthesis, $_m$RNA synthesis
      Catabolic—Inhibits gluconeogenesis. Increases glucose oxidation
      Other—Increases transport glucose and A.A. across cell membrane (does not affect glucose entrance into hepatic cells, brain, blood cells). Inhibits cyclic AMP formation

Organismal

Inhibits mobilization of fat from peripheral reservoirs

Decreases blood (sugar, K, PO_4 ketones), liver gluconeogenesis, polyuria

Increases liver and muscle glycogen, glucose absorption in gut, fat formation, nitrogen balance

9. Catabolism

Intermediates—Insulinase in liver (antagonized by insulinase inhibitor)

Excretion products—Metabolic products of amino acids

MISCELLANEOUS

1. **Relationship to Vitamins:**   Vitamin C acts similarly to alloxan (i.e., antagonist)

2. **Relationship to Other Hormones**

Cortisol, Glucagon, Epinephrine, Norepinephrine, T4, STH (CHO and fat metabolism)—Antagonistic to insulin

Estradiol, Testosterone, STH (protein metabolism)—Synergistic with insulin

3. **Unusual Features**

Contains 0.4% zinc in crystals

First synthetic polypeptide hormone

Multiple insulins in rat, bonito

Forms fibrils when heated at low pH

Antibody sites not identical with biological activity sites

Frog—Pancreas not active until mid-metamorphosis

Urodeles—Only β-cells in pancreas

Vigorous exercise increases rate of transport of glucose into muscle cells even in absence of insulin

4. **Possible Relationships of Deficiency Symptoms to Metabolic Action**

Hyperglycemia, decrease in respiratory quotient—Inability to metabolize and transport glucose into cells

Hyperlipemia—Mobilization of fat from peripheral reserves

Ketonemia—Incomplete oxidation of mobilized fat

Azoturia (decrease in tissue protein)—Induced gluconeogenesis producing urea and ammonia

Polydipsia—Thirst produced by glycosuria (polyuria)

Polyphagia—Hunger produced by loss of urinary glucose

30
Glucagon

GENERAL INFORMATION

1. **Synonyms:** HGF, HG-Factor, hyperglycemic-glycogenolytic factor, glukagon

2. **History**

   1922—McLeod ⎤
   1923—Collip ⎦ Described hyperglycemic effect of pancreatic extracts

   1923—Kimball and Murlin suggested a second pancreatic hormone; named it glucagon

   1955—Staub, Sinn, and Behrens isolated and crystallized glucagon

   1956—Bromer *et al.* determined structure of glucagon

   1967—Wunsch synthesized glucagon

3. **Physiological Forms:** *l*-glucagon

4. **Active Analogs and Related Compounds:** Serotonin (G.I. tract, spleen, skin, tongue); isoproterenol, G.I. glucagon

5. **Inactive Analogs and Related Compounds:** UV-inactivated glucagon

6. **Antagonists:** Insulin

7. **Synergists:** Epinephrine (liver, muscle), norepinephrine, cortisol, cortisone

8. **Physiological Functions**

Increases—Blood sugar, blood K^+, O_2 consumption, liver glycogenolysis, gluconeogenesis, nitrogen and salt excretion, glucose-1-P

Decreases—Liver glycogen, protein formation, gastric juice, fatty acid synthesis

9. **Deficiency Diseases, Disorders:**   Hypoglycemic coma

10. **Essentiality for Life:**   Not essential for life of vertebrate organisms

CHEMISTRY

1. **Structure**

Polypeptide (sequence determined): His—Ser—Glu—Gly—Thr—Phe—Thr—Ser—Asp—Tyr—Ser—Lys—Tyr—Leu—Asp—Ser—Arg—Arg—Ala—Glu—Asp—Phe—Val—Glu—Try—Leu—Met—Asp—Thr

Straight single chain—His. - - - Thr., 29 amino acids

No S—S bridges

2. **Reactions**

Heat—Stable to 100°C

Acid—Stable, pH 2

Alkali—Stable, pH 9

Water—Sol., basic

Oxidation—No data

Reduction—Stable to cysteine (removes contaminating insulin)

Light—UV Inactivates

Proteolysis—Leucine amino peptidase, pepsin, trypsin, chymotrypsin at pH = 6-8 hydrolyze

3. **Properties**

Appearance—White powder

MW—3500 (29 A.A.)

MP—No data

Crystal Form—Rhombic dodecahedra

Salts—HCl

Important Groups for Activity Try, Met

Solubility

H_2O—Insol.

Acet., Alc.—Insol.

Benz., Chl., Eth.—Insol.

Absn. Max.—278 mμ

Chemical Nature—Basic polypeptide

Misc.—pI = 7.5-8.5

4. **Commercial Production:**   Hog pancreas

5. Isolation
    Sources—Crude pork insulin
    Methods
        Ppt. with acetone and salts at low pH
        Crystallize from 0.033 M glycine buffer. pH 8.6 with 0.67 M urea
        Purification: Starch zone electrophoresis

6. Determination
    Bioassay
        Hyperglycemic response in cats
        Glycogenolysis of liver slices
        Reaction of phosphorylase in liver slices
    Physicochemical—Radioimmunoassay, immunoassay

MEDICAL AND BIOLOGICAL ROLE

1. **Species Occurrence, Specificity, and Antigenicity**
    Occurrence—Found in fish through mammals
    Specificity—Interspecies potency—Interreactive
    Antigenicity—Antigenic in rabbit or bovine x porcine glucagon, but not
        guinea pig glucagon

2. **Units:**   By weight, also 1 I.U. = amount to increase blood sugar to
        30 mg/100 ml

3. **Normal Blood Levels (Man):**   0.02-0.05 μg/100 ml plasma

4. **Administration**
    Injection—Glucagon HCl intravenous, intramuscular, or subcutaneous
        Used to treat insulin-induced hypoglycemia
    Topical—Inactive
    Oral—Inactive

5. **Factors Affecting Release**
    Inhibitors—High blood sugar, $CoCl_2$ (α-cells)
    Stimulators—Hypoglycemia, fasting

6. **Deficiency Symptoms:**   Low blood glucose

7. **Effects of Overdose:**   Metaglucagon diabetes (destroy β-cells), increased
        food consumption, high blood glucose

METABOLIC ROLE

1. **Biosynthesis**

   Simple precursors—16 of standard 20 amino acids (no cysteine, isoleucine, proline, glutamic acid)

   Intermediates—Unknown

   Site(s) in cell—No data

2. **Production Sites**—α-cells in pancreas

3. **Storage Areas:**   Granules in α-cells

4. **Blood Carriers:**   Plasma proteins

5. **Half-life:**   Less than 10 min

6. **Target Tissues:**   Liver, adipose tissues, kidney

7. **Reactions**

   Reactive intermediate—Cyclic AMP—secondary messenger

Organ	Enzyme System	Effect
Liver	Glucokinase	Inhibited
	Glycogen synthetase	Inhibited
	Glycogenolysis enzymes	Activated
	Gluconeogenesis enzymes	Activated
	Adenyl cyclase	Activated
	Dephosphophosphorylase kinase	Activated
	Phosphorylase b	Activated
	Carbamoyl phosphate synthetase	Activated
	Argino-succinase	Activated
	Argino-succinic synthetase	Activated
Heart	Adenyl cyclase	Activated

8. **Mode of Action**

   Cellular

   Anabolic—No data

   Catabolic

   Decreased protein and fatty acid synthesis

   Increased lipolysis

   Increased CHO glycogenolysis

   Increased protein catabolism

   Other

   Increased cyclic AMP formation

   Decreased adrenal ascorbic acid

Organismal
Stimulates hepatic glycogenolysis and gluconeogenesis
Increases adipose tissue lipolysis
Stimulates release of catecholamines by adrenal medulla
Increases nitrogen K, Na, Cl, PO_4 excretion
Increases blood sugar, ketone bodies
Decreases gastric juice flow
Increases heart rate, ventricular contractility
Decreases atrio-ventricular conduction time
Retards G.I. contractions

9. Catabolism

Intermediates—Proteolysis in liver, kidney, blood—glucagonase (protease), recycling
Excretion products—End products of protein metabolism (urea, CO_2)

MISCELLANEOUS

1. Relationship to Vitamins
Vitamin C—Depletion of adrenal ascorbic acid by glucagon

2. Relationship to Other Hormones
Epinephrine, Norepinephrine—Secretion stimulated by glucagon, also synergistic
Cortisol, Cortisone—Synergistic to glucagon
Insulin—Antagonistic to glucagon

3. Unusual Features
Tissue differences in glucagon response
More conc. in female than male pancreas
G.I. glucagon not identical with pancreatic glucagon
Traces of heavy metals (Cu, Co) found in glucagon preparations

4. Possible Relationships of Deficiency Symptoms to Metabolic Action
Low blood glucose—lack of glucose-releasing activity by glucagon into plasma

31
Aldosterone

GENERAL INFORMATION

1. **Synonyms:** Electrocortin, mineralocorticoid, aldocortin, 18-oxocorticosterone

2. **History**

   1953—Simpson *et al.* ⎫ Isolated crystalline aldosterone
   1954—Mattox *et al.* ⎭ from adrenals
   1954—Wettstein and Anner devised highly sensitive test for mineralocorticoid activity
   1954—Simpson *et al.* determined structure of aldosterone
   1955—Schmidlin *et al.* synthesized dl-aldosterone
   1956—Vischer *et al.* synthesized d-aldosterone
   1956—Neher and Wettstein isolated 15 more steroids similar to aldosterone and cortisol

3. **Physiological Forms:** Hemiacetal form (11,18-semiacetal), aldehyde form

4. **Active Analogs and Related Forms** (Mineralocorticoids)
   Natural—11-Deoxycorticosterone, corticosterone
   Synthetic—2α-Methylcortisol, 9α-fluorocortisol, 2α-methyl-9α-fluorocortisol

5. **Inactive Analogs and Related Forms (for Aldosterone Function):** Cortexolone, dexamethasone, prednisolone

6. **Antagonists**
   Natural—Cortisol, pineal factor, estradiol, progesterone, vasopressin (kidney), prostaglandins
   Synthetic—3-Spironolactone, aldactone-A

7. **Synergists:**   11-deoxycorticosterone, vasopressin, oxytocin, angiotensin II, renin, STH

8. **Physiological Functions**
   Maintenance of normal electrolyte blood balance
   Prolongs survival of adrenalectomized animals
   Accelerates gluconeogenesis
   Regulates kidney function

9. **Deficiency Diseases, Disorders:**   Addison's disease, (deficiency), Cushing's syndrome (excess), adrenocortical insufficiency, primary hyper-aldosteronism

10. **Essentiality for Life:**   One of the most essential of all hormones. Absence can be fatal in short time period

CHEMISTRY

1. **Structure**

Aldosterone (aldehyde form), $C_{21}H_{28}O_5$

2. **Reactions**

Heat—Stable
Acid—Decomposes
Alkali—Fluoresces (conc.)
   Isomerizes to 17-iso-aldosterone
Water—Slightly sol.

Oxidation—Loses aldehyde group
Reduction—Unstable
Light—Stable

3. **Properties**

Appearance—Colorless crystals	Solubility
MW—360.4	H_2O—Sparingly
MP—164°C	Acet., Alc.—Sol.
Crystal Form—Needles (acetate)	Benz., Chl., Eth.—Sol.
Salts, Esters—Acetate	Absn. Max.—240 mμ
Important Groups for Activity	Chemical Nature
—C(18)HO	Hemiacetal, aldehyde
—C(21)H$_2$OH	Alc., ketone—Reducing steroid
—C(11)OH	α_D^{23} = +145 (acet.)

4. **Commercial Production:**   Microbiological (stereospecific hydroxylation)

5. **Isolation**

Sources: Beef adrenal extract

Methods
   (1) Partition aqueous extract with pentane-methanol
   (2) Chromatograph on kieselguhr, elute with petroleum ether-benzene-$CHCl_3$
   (3) Rechromatograph on powdered cellulose, elution with toluene-petroleum ether-methanol
   (4) Recrystallize from methanol

6. **Determination**

Bioassay
   Life maintenance in adrenalectomized animals
   Increase muscular work performance
   Cold stress reactions on adrenalectomy
   In vitro incubation of perfused tissues
   Physicochemical—Monitor Na/K ratios in urine

MEDICAL AND BIOLOGICAL ROLE

1. **Species Occurrence, Specificity, and Antigenicity**
   Occurrence: All vertebrate species studied, except cyclostomes
   Specificity: Same electrolyte regulator, all species
   Antigenicity: None reported

2. **Units:**   mg or μg

3. **Normal Blood Levels (Man):**   0.03 μg/100 ml

4. Administration
    Injection—Main route
    Topical—No reports
    Oral—Active

5. Factors Affecting Release
    Inhibitors
        Decreased K^+ in blood
        Increased Na^+ in blood
        Hemodilution
    Stimulators
        Angiotensin II—Renin
        Stress, decreased Na^+, decreased blood vol.
        Pregnancy
        ACTH (slightly)
        Increased blood pressure in carotid arteries
        Increased K^+ in blood

6. Deficiency Symptoms (Humans)
    Decreased—Blood (pressure, sugar, pH), weight, liver glycogen, urinary
        K^+, temperature, reproductive functions
    Increased—Urinary (Na^+, Cl^-, HCO_3^-)
    Kidney failure, muscular weakness, GI disturbances, hemoconcentration,
        stress intolerance, acidosis

7. Effects of Overdose, Excess
    Hypertension
    Congestive heart failure
    Increased Na^+ and H_2O in blood, muscles
    Hemodilution
    Hypokalemia
    Edema
    Alkalosis
    Diabetes insipidus (type of)

METABOLIC ROLE

1. **Biosynthesis:**   Acetate → Mevalonate → Squalene → Cholesterol → Preg-
        nenolone → Progesterone → Aldosterone
    Site(s) in Cell—Membranes

2. **Production Sites:**   Adrenal cortex (zona glomerulosa), embryonic rest cells

3. **Storage Areas:**   None

4. **Blood Carriers**
    Lipoproteins, albumin
    Conjugates, Free Steroid—Combined with above proteins

5. **Half-life:**   25 min

6. **Target Tissues:**   Distal renal tubules, sweat and salivary glands, intestinal mucosa, gills (fish), skin (amphibia), nasal gland (bird), rectal gland (sharks)

7. **Reactions**
    Reactive form—Equilibrium (hemiacetal-aldehyde) redox couple

Organ	Enzyme System	Effect
Kidney	1. Unknown enzymes involved in sodium transport	Activated
	2. Also enzymes similar to cortisol (glucocorticoid function)	Activated
	3. RNA polymerase	Activated
Liver, muscle, plasma, general	Similar to cortisol; see Cortisol	Activated

8. **Mode of Action**
    Cellular
        Anabolic—Liver (proteins, CHO, nucleic acids)
        Catabolic—Extrahepatic (proteins, fats, CHO, nucleic acids)
        Other—Increases Na^+ active transport in renal tubules, activates redox pump, H_2O transported with Na^+
    Organismal
        Increases blood Na^+, volume, pressure; urinary K^+, H^+; cold tolerance, muscle work performance, liver glycogen
        Decreases blood K^+, H^+; urine Na^+, H_2O, volume; eosinophils, lymphocytes

9. **Catabolism**
    Intermediates—Tetrahydro derivative (inactive)
    Excretion Products—30-40% Glucuronides, 4-8% free, 52-66% other conjugates

MISCELLANEOUS

1. **Relationship to Vitamins**

   Vitamin C—Adrenal cortex depleted of vit. C on production of aldosterone

   Niacin—NADPH involved in synthesis of aldosterone

   Biotin—Prolongs life in adrenalectomized rats

2. **Relationship to Other Hormones**

   Cortisol—Synergistic to aldosterone in glucocorticoid activity; antagonistic to aldosterone in water metabolism

   ACTH—Trigger for small release of aldosterone

   Vasopressin, Oxytocin—Synergists for aldosterone action in water metabolism

   Angiotensin II, Renin—Stimulate production of aldosterone

   Other hormones antagonistic or synergistic with cortisol (glucocorticoid action)—*see* Cortisol

3. **Unusual Features**

   Not a glucocorticoid even though it has —OH on C-11 and 1/3 of glucocorticoid power of cortisol

   Redox couple—Hemiacetal-aldehyde equilibrium

   No nervous controls

   Active on oral administration

   Most water soluble of all steroids

   Largely independent of ACTH control

4. **Possible Relationships of Deficiency Symptoms to Metabolic Action**

   Loss of mineralocorticoid functions. Failure of sodium pump and sodium-water reabsorption mechanisms in kidney tubules

   Increased—Urinary (Na^+, Cl^-, HCO_3^-). Decreased urinary K^+, blood pH and pressure

   Acidosis, kidney failure

   Hemoconcentration

   Weight loss

   Loss of glucocorticoid functions; decreased gluconeogenesis

   Muscular weakness

   G.I. disturbances

   Stress intolerance

   Decreased blood sugar

   Decreased liver glycogen

   Decreased temperature

32
Cortisol

GENERAL INFORMATION

1. **Synonyms:** Hydrocortisone, Compound F, 17-hydroxycorticosterone, Substance M

2. **History**
   1937—Reichstein isolated cortisol from adrenal glands
   1942—Von Euw, Reichstein determined configuration of cortisol
   1948—Mason, Sprague isolated cortisol from urine
   1950—Reich *et al.* isolated cortisol from blood
   1950—Wendler *et al.* synthesized cortisol
   1951—Zaffaroni *et al.* demonstrated biosynthesis of cortisol in adrenals

3. **Physiological Forms:** Cortisol, cortisone

4. **Active Analogs and Related Compounds (Glucocorticoids)**
   Natural—Deoxycorticosterone, cortexolone, cortisone ("E"), corti costerone ("B"), dehydrocorticosterone ("A")
   Synthetic—Dexamethasone, 9α-F-cortisol, prednisone, prednisolone

5. **Inactive Analogs and Related Compounds:** Estrone, progesterone, 17-α-hydroxyprogesterone, cortexolone, adrenosterone

6. **Antagonists:** Protein and CHO metabolism—Insulin; STH, estrogens, testosterone

7. **Synergists:** Fat metabolism—STH; epinephrine, norepinephrine, PTH, T4

8. **Physiological Functions**

Increases—Protein catabolism (exc. liver) gluconeogensis, carbohydrate anabolism (liver), blood sugar, glucose absorption, brain excitation, spread of infections, urinary glucose and nitrogen, stress tolerance, lactation, water diuresis

Decreases—Fat anabolism, growth rate, inflammation, eosinophils, lymphocytes, antigen sensitivity, respiratory quotient, ketosis, wound healing, skin pigmentation, RBC hemolysis

Regulates—General adaptation syndrome, water balance, blood pressure, hormone release

9. **Disorders and Deficiency Diseases:** Addison's disease (deficiency), Cushing's syndrome (excess), adrenal insufficiency, adrenogenital syndrome, rheumatic arthritis, inflammation

10. **Essentiality for Life:** Absence causes shortening of life span due to inability to respond to stress situations

CHEMISTRY

1. **Structure:**

Cortisol, $C_{21}H_{30}O_5$

2. **Reactions**

Heat—Oxidizes	Oxidation—Forms cortisone
Acid—Esterifies	C-11 Hydroxyl $\rightarrow$ Keto
Fluorescent in H_2SO_4 (conc.)	Reduction—Stable
Alkali—Stable (dilute)	Light—Stable
Fluorescent (conc.)	
Water—very sl. sol.	

3. Properties

Appearance—White powder
MW—362.5
MP—217-220°C
Crystal Form—Rectilinear
  plates
Salts, Esters—
  Acetate
Important Groups for Activity
  —C(17)OH
  —C(11)OH
  —C(21)H$_2$OH

Solubility
  H$_2$O—0.28 mg/ml
  Acet., Alc.—15, 6.2 mg/ml
  Chl., Eth.—9.3, 0.35 mg/ml
  Absn. Max.—242 mμ
Chemical Nature
  Reducing agent
  Alcohol, ketone
  α_D^{22} = 167 (EtOH)

4. Commercial Production: Extraction and isolation from beef and hog adrenals

5. Isolation

Sources—Adrenal cortex
Methods
  Free
    Extract with dil. alkali, partition between 2 solvents
    Chromatography—Glass, paper, thin layer, gas, liquid
    Columns—Florasil
    Countercurrent distribution
  Conjugates—Extract tissue, paper chromatography, alumina columns

6. Determination

Bioassay:
  Increased—Liver glycogen, lifespan in cold, tolerance to trauma,
    isotope uptake.
  Decreased—Eosinophils, lymphocytes
Physicochemical
  Reduction to red formazan
  Oxidation to 17-oxosteroids
  Phenylhydrazone formation
  Fluorescence at 550 or 570 mμ
  Polarography

MEDICAL AND BIOLOGICAL ROLE

1. **Species Occurrence, Specificity, and Antigenicity**
   Occurrence—Cortisol major form of glucocorticoids in primates, dog, fish, decreasing in activity in lower forms. Corticosterone major glucocorticoid in rodents, birds, amphibians, reptiles
   Specificity—Can cross species lines without loss of activity
   Antigenicity—Not antigenic

2. **Units:**   By weight, μg

3. **Normal Blood Levels:**   10 μg/100 ml (man)

4. **Administration**
   Injection—Intramuscular
   Oral—Active. Prednisone form used
   Topical—Acetonides in creams, lotions

5. **Factors Affecting Release**
   Inhibitors
       Pituitary hypofunction
       Diurnal rhythm—Low in afternoon
       Decreased ACTH
       Increased plasma-glucocorticoids
   Stimulators
       Pregnancy, infancy, stress
       ACTH ingestion and ACTH increase
       Adrenal hyperfunction
       Angiotensin II, insulin, estrogens
       Glucagon, vasopressin
       Decreased plasma glucocorticoids

6. **Deficiency Symptoms (Humans)**
   Decreased
       Growth, secondary sex characteristics
       Blood pressure, body temperature
       Kidney function, leading to death
       Liver glycogen, gluconeogenesis
       Intestinal absorption, blood sugar
       Stress response—ultimately death
   Increased
       Glucose oxidation, ACTH levels, respiratory quotient

Fat anabolism, hemoconcentration
Muscular weakness
Skin pigmentation
Insulin sensitivity

7. **Effects of Overdose (Excess)**
Buffalo obesity, bruisability, moon-face
Osteoporosis (demineralization of bone)
Adrenal regression
Anesthesia
Atherosclerosis, hypercholesterolemia, lipemia
Diabetes
Alkalosis
Decreased growth
Inhibition of inflammatory responses and wound healing

METABOLIC ROLE

1. **Biosynthesis:**   Acetate $\rightarrow$ Mevalonate $\rightarrow$ Squalene $\rightarrow$ Cholesterol
$\rightarrow$ Pregnenolone $\rightarrow$ Progesterone $\rightarrow$ 17α-Hydroxyprogesterone
$\rightarrow$ Cortisol
Sites in cell—Mitochondria, microsomes

2. **Production Sites:**   Adrenal cortex, placenta, embryonic rest cells

3. **Storage:**   Adrenal cortex (small amount)

4. **Blood Carriers:**   Lipoproteins, conjugates, α-globulins (transcortin), albumin; also free

5. **Half-life:**   1½-3 hr

6. **Target Tissues:**   Liver, central nervous system, hypothalamus, thymus, lymph nodes, intestine, connective tissues, skin, mammary gland, vascular system, general systemic

7. **Reactions**
Reactive Form: Cortisol $\rightleftharpoons$ cortisone (redox couple)

Enzyme Systems:

Organ	Enzyme Systems	Effect
Liver	Phosphoenolpyruvate carboxykinase	Activated
	Pyruvate carboxylase	Activated
	Tryptophan pyrrolase	Activated
	Glycolytic cycle enzymes	Activated
	Krebs cycle enzymes	Activated
	Urea cycle enzymes	Activated
	Deaminases and transaminases	Activated
Liver, kidney	Glucose-6-phosphatase	Activated
	Glycogen synthetase	Activated
	Arginase	Activated
Liver, plasma	Alkaline phosphatase	Activated
Muscle	Aminopeptidase	Activated
General	Histidine decarboxylase	Inhibited
	Hexokinase	Inhibited

8. Mode of Action

Cellular

Anabolic—Increases liver (protein, nucleic acid, CHO, fat) synthesis

Catabolic—Increases extrahepatic (protein, lipid, and nucleic acid) breakdown; decreases extrahepatic CHO breakdown

Other—Redox mechanisms maintained; water and sodium membrane transport regulated in kidney glomerulus (with aldosterone)

Organismal

Maintains circulation and blood pressure (with aldosterone)

Maintains fluid balance (with aldosterone)

Maintains renal function (with aldosterone)

Releases other hormones

Maintains stress reactions

Regulates ACTH output of pituitary

Maintains collagen, capillary permeability

9. Catabolism

Intermediates—Bile salts, 17-hydroxy steroids

Excretion products

Urine

100 (approx.) different steroids in urine

87% Glucuronides or sulfates—Cortols, cortolones, 17-hydroxy steroids

4% Free metabolites—Cortols, cortolones, 17-hydroxy steroids

1% Free cortisol—Cortols, cortolones, 17-hydroxy steroids

Feces—Bile salt derivatives

MISCELLANEOUS

1. **Relationship to Vitamins**

    Vitamin C—May be needed for steroid hormone biosynthesis; depleted from adrenal cortex on cortical secretion

    Niacin—NADPH required for steroid hormone biosynthesis

    Vitamin D—Action antagonized by cortisol, i.e., reduces Ca absorption in intestine

    Pantothenic acid, folic acid maintain secretions of steroids by adrenal cortex

    Biotin—Adrenocortical insufficiency noted in biotin deficiency

    Vitamin A—Deficiency of vitamin A causes cortical necrosis

2. **Relationship to Other Hormones**

    Estradiol-17β—Antagonist to cortisol protein metabolic effects

    Insulin—Antagonist to cortisol (CHO, protein, lipid) metabolic effects

    STH—Antagonist to cortisol protein metabolic effects

    Testosterone—Antagonist to cortisol protein metabolic effects

    Cortisone—Converted to cortisol in body (redox couple)

    T4, Norepinephrine, Epinephrine—Potentiated by cortisol, synergistic

    ACTH—Production stopped via feedback mechanism of cortisol

    PTH—Synergist to cortisol in bone resorption

    Vasopressin, Oxytocin—Antagonist to cortisol water balance effects, stimulants for production of glucocorticoids

    Glucagon—Stimulant for production of cortical hormones

3. **Unusual Features**

    Production of euphoria, anesthetic action

    Decreased activity if side chain is lengthened

    Substituents on C-20, C-18, determine antihemolytic activity

    Suppression of mast cell activity, migration of lymphocytes and phagocytes

    Inhibition of wound healing and collagen formation by fibroblasts

    Inhibition of antibody production, regression of thymus tissue

    Suppresses mitosis in lymphoid tissue

    Species difference in sensitivity

4. **Possible Relationships of Deficiency Symptoms to Metabolic Action**

    Osteoporosis—Antagonism to vit. D; synergism with PTH

    Diabetes—Inhibition of glucose oxidation

    Alkalosis—Retention of sodium

    Bruisability—Depletion of vit. C (?)

Buffalo obesity, Moon-face—Antagonism to insulin (?)
Adrenal regression—Shut-off of ACTH production
Anesthesia—Effects on membranes (?)
Atherosclerosis—Diabetogenic effect (?)

33
Estradiol

GENERAL INFORMATION

1. **Synonyms:** Estradiol-17β, female hormone, β-estradiol, dihydrotheelin, dihydrofollicular hormone, dihydrofolliculin

2. **History**
   1929—Doisy, Butenandt, *et al.* isolated and crystallized estrone from pregnancy urine
   1930—Marrian isolated estriol from pregnancy urine
   1932—Marrian, Butenandt determined structure of estrone and estriol
   1936—McCorquodale isolated crystalline estradiol from pregnancy urine and sow ovaries
   1940—Inhoffen synthesized estradiol from cholesterol
   1948—Anner and Miescher totally synthesized estrone

3. **Physiological Forms:** Estrone, estriol, estradiol (Estrogens)

4. **Active Analogs and Related Compounds** (Estrogens)
   Synthetic—Diethylstilbesterol, hexestrol, dienestrol, benzestrol, ethinyl-estradiol, chlorotrianisene
   Natural—Estriol, estrone, equilin

5. **Inactive Analogs and Related Compounds** (Estrogen function)
   Pregnanediol, lumiestrone, progesterone, 17α-estradiol, 17α-hydroxy-progesterone, 17α-hydroxypregnenolone

6. **Antagonists:**   Progesterone, cortisol, testosterone (all concentration dependent); uterine factor, melatonin, ethamoxytriphetol, aldosterone

7. **Synergists:**   Prolactin, progesterone, androgens, corticoids, STH, oxytocin, T4, relaxin, insulin

8. **Physiological Functions**
   Regulates menstrual cycle, female sex behavior
   Maintains secondary sex characteristics
   Affects antibody properties
   Induces estrus, uterine hypertrophy, vaginal cornification, potentiates and stimulates calcitonin secretion

9. **Deficiency Diseases, Disorders:**   Menopause (natural deficiency) gonadal dysgenesis, delayed maturation

10. **Essentiality for Life:**   Not for life of organism, but for reproduction of organism

CHEMISTRY

1. **Structure**

Estradiol-17β, $C_{18}H_{24}O_2$

2. **Reactions**

Heat—Stable	Oxidation—Unstable. Forms
Acid—Stable (dilute)	estriol or estrone
Fluoresces (conc.)	Reduction—Unstable
Alkali—Sol., stable	Light—No data
Water—Insol.	

3. **Properties**

Appearance—colorless powder	MP—173-179°C
MW—272.4	Crystal Form—Prisms

Salts, Esters—Acetate, benzoate, propionate, heptanoate, valerate

Important Groups for Activity

Aromatic Ring A

−C(3)OH, −C(17)OH

Solubility

H_2O—Insol.

(Estriol—3 mg/100 cc H_2O)

Acet., Alc.—Sol.

Benz., Chl., Eth.—Sol.

Absn. Max.—225, 280 mμ

Chemical Nature—Alcohol, aromatic, phenolic

α_D^{22} = 76-83

4. **Commercial Production**

Extract pregnant mare's urine

Total synthesis

5. **Isolation**

Sources—Pregnancy urine of mares, follicular liquor of sow ovaries

Method

Protein-bound or conjugated steroids: 15% HCl, 60 min 100°C, or sephadex G-25 with H_2O elution, or amberlite column LA-2, elution with ethyl acetate at pH = 2; saponification

Free steroids: ether extraction

Purification

Countercurrent distribution

Column chromatography

High-voltage electrophoresis

6. **Determination**

Bioassay

Vaginal cornification

Increase in uterine weight in ovariectomized animals

Topical application in vagina; vaginal smear of exfoliated cells

Physicochemical

Fluorescence assay

Colorimetry—Kober reaction

Chromatography

Radioimmunoassay

MEDICAL AND BIOLOGICAL ROLE

1. **Species Occurrence, Specificity, Antigenicity**

Occurrence—All vertebrates, but different distribution of activities for three physiological forms. Some plants

Specificity
    17β-Estradiol, estrone (human, dog, pig, rat)
    Estrone, equilin, equilinin (horse)
    17α-Estradiol (sheep, goat, beef)
    17-Epiestriol (mouse)
    Species difference in sensitivity
Antigenicity—No antigenicity reported

2. Units: 1 mg = 10,000 I.U.

3. Normal Blood Levels (Man): Male .008 μg/100 ml (estradiol and estrone). Females 0.2 μg/100 ml or less (estrone and estriol). Pregnant Females (av.) 2.1 μg/100 ml estradiol, 6.5 μg/100 ml estrone, 10.9 μg/100 ml estriol (varies with stage of pregnancy)

4. Administration:
    Injection—Subcutaneous, intramuscular
    Topical—In creams and cosmetics
    Oral—Inactive free form. Active as esters or synthetic analogs. Various synthetic estrogens used in small quantity with synthetic progestogens in contraceptive pills

5. Factors Affecting Release
    Inhibitors—Feedback via blood to hypothalamus
    Stimulators—FSH and LH (cyclic via hypothalamus)

6. Deficiency Symptoms (Humans)
    Delayed maturation
    Female accessory and reproductive organs regress
    Decreased female behavioral pattern
    Senescence
    Menopause

7. Effects of Overdose, Excess
    Tumors
    Inhibition of gonads (decrease FSH, LH) → permanent sterility

METABOLIC ROLE

1. Biosynthesis: Acetate → Mevalonate → Squalene → Cholesterol
    → Pregnenolone → Progesterone → 17α-Hydroxyprogesterone
    → Androstenedione → Testosterone → 19-Hydroxytestosterone
    → Estradiol
Site(s) in cell—Mitochondria, microsomes

2. **Production Sites**
All vertebrates
Ovarian follicles (membrane granulosa, theca interna)
Testes (interstitial cells)
Corpus luteum, adrenal cortex (fasciculata reticularis)
Placenta, embryonic rest cells

3. **Storage Areas:**   Unknown

4. **Blood Carriers**
Plasma proteins—Estriol glucuronides, free estrone and estradiol
Plasma lipoprotein, estroprotein, serum albumin, red cell proteins

5. **Half-life:**   2-4 min

6. **Target Tissues:**   Systemic; uterus, mammary gland, vagina, ovary (corpus luteum), secondary female sex organs, skin, CNS, thyroid, thymus, long bones, anterior pituitary, hypothalamus

7. **Reactions**
Reactive forms (Redox couple)
Estradiol $\rightleftharpoons$ estrone $\rightarrow$ estriol (oxidation product)

Organ	Enzyme System	Effect
Uterus	Lactic acid dehydrogenase	Activated
	Phosphorylase b $\rightarrow$ a	Activated
	RNA polymerase	Activated
Placenta	Isocitric dehydrogenase	Activated
Endometrium	Glucose-6-phosphate dehydrogenase	Activated
Kidney	Kynurenine aminotransferase	Inhibited
Liver	Kynureninase	Inhibited
	N^l-Methylnicotinamide oxidase	Inhibited

8. **Mode of Action**
Cellular
Anabolic
RNA and protein synthesis (uterus) increased
CHO synthesis (uterus) increased
Increased growth (uterus)
Catabolic—CHO glycolysis (uterus) increased
Other
Direct action on nucleus

Increases mitosis (uterus)
Transcription of RNA affected
Hyperpolarization of cell membranes
Organismal
Uterus
Increases glycolysis, respiration, H_2O permeability, hyperemia
Releases histamine
Potentiates and stimulates TCT in calcium bone deposition
Development of female characteristics
Growth of female $1°$ and $2°$ sex organs
Estradiol, estrone—Act on corpus luteum
Estriol—Acts on sex organs
Regulates menstrual cycle and sex behavior
Maintains secondary sex characteristics
Affects antibody properties

9. **Catabolism**
Intermediates—Estriol
Excretion Products

Urine—Mainly conjugated $\dfrac{\text{estrone glucuronide or } SO_4}{\text{estriol glucuronide or } SO_4} = 1/3$

Free—As estriol or 16-epiestriol
Pregnancy—Estrone + estradiol increases 100x. Estriol increases 1000x
Feces—Enterohepatic circulation of estrogens

MISCELLANEOUS

1. **Relationship to Vitamins**
Folic acid—Involved in mitotic effect of estradiol
Niacin (TPN)(DPN)—Involved in increased respiration and in cholesterol precursor synthesis
Vitamin E—Involved in gonadotropin production or release
Vitamin B_6—Competes as cofactor with estrogen sulfate in kynurenine aminotransferase activity
Vitamin D—Synergistic in calcium metabolism with estradiol

2. **Relationship to Other Hormones**
Progesterone, Cortisol, Testosterone—Antagonistic or synergistic to estradiol depending on relative concentrations of estradiol and other hormone

Prolactin, STH, Oxytocin, T4, Relaxin—Synergistic to estradiol
TCT—Potentiated and stimulated by estradiol
FSH, LH—Stimulate release or production of estradiol

3. Unusual Features

Estradiol-17β $\rightleftharpoons$ estrone $\rightarrow$ estriol (activity 1000:100:1)
Aromatic ring—Carcinogenicity implicated
Redox couple estradiol $\rightleftharpoons$ estrone
Derived from testosterone in biosynthesis
Occurrence of estrogens in plants—Genistein, Coumestrol (active)
Tumor formation enhanced by estradiol
Enterohepatic circulation of estradiol
Variable species forms
Synthetic estrogens not steroids

4. Possible Relationships of Deficiency to Metabolic Action

Ovarian regression—Decrease of mitosis in sex tissues
Regression of female sex organs and secondary sex characteristics—
decrease of mitosis in sex tissues
Decreased female sex behavior patterns—Decrease of estradiol in central
nervous system.
Senescence, menopause—Decrease in mitosis in sex organs

34
Progesterone

GENERAL INFORMATION

1. **Synonyms:**   Progestin, luteosterone, corpus luteum hormone

2. **History**
    1903—Fraenkel demonstrated that removal of corpora lutea in pregnant rabbits terminates pregnancy, prevents attachment of ovum to uterus
    1928—Corner and Allen restored progestational changes in above rabbits with extracts of corpora lutea
    1930—Fels and Slotta ⎫
    1932—Allen ⎬ Obtained crude crystalline concentrates
    1932—Fevold and Hisaw ⎭ containing progestational activity
    1934—Butenandt et al. ⎫
         Slotta et al. ⎬ Isolated pure crystalline
         Allen et al. ⎪ corpus luteum hormone
         Hartmann et al. ⎭
    1934—Slotta et al. proposed formula for corpus luteum hormone
    1934—Butenandt, Fernholz synthesized progesterone from stigmasterol

3. **Physiological Forms:**   Progesterone, 17α-Hydroxyprogesterone

4. **Active Analogs and Related Compounds:**   (Progestins, progestogens)
    Natural
        20α-Hydroxypregnenone

20β-Hydroxypregnenone
11-Dehydroprogesterone
Cortexone
17α-Hydroxyprogesterone
Synthetic
A-Norprogesterone
19-Norprogesterone
21-Norprogesterone
Ethisterone
17α-Methyltestosterone
6α-Methyl-17α-acetoxyprogesterone
Δ^1-Dehydro-6α-methyl-17α-acetoxyprogesterone

5. **Inactive Analogs and Related Compounds**
   5α-Pregnane-3β-ol-20-one, 21-ethylprogesterone
   11β-Hydroxyprogesterone, pregnanediol, pregnanetriol

6. **Antagonists:**   (Estradiol, testosterone, oxytocin, aldosterone) all concentration dependent

7. **Synergists:**   Estradiol, prolactin, testosterone, cortisol, STH, T4, relaxin, oxytocin

8. **Physiological Functions**
   Low concentrations
      Prepare uterus for blastocyst implantation, promote ovulation and mammary gland development
      Regulate female sex accessory organs, weak corticosteroid properties, precursor to sex hormones
   Higher concentrations
      Maintain pregnancy, repress ovulation and sex activity, inhibit vaginal cornification, and parturition, decrease myometrial excitation

9. **Deficiency Diseases, Disorders:**   Pseudopregnancy (laboratory animals), acne, dysfunctional uterine bleeding

10. **Essentiality for Life**
    Indirectly essential for life via corticosteroid requirement
    Essential for aldosterone and glucocorticoid formation
    Essential for reproduction in female vertebrates

CHEMISTRY

Structure

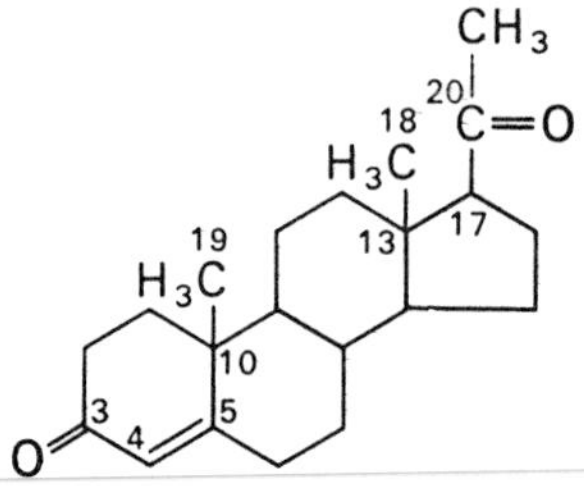

Progesterone, $C_{21}H_{30}O_2$

2. Reactions

Heat—Stable	Oxidation—Unstable
Acid—Unstable; fluoresces in H_2SO_4	Reduction—Unstable; reduces to pregnanediol
Alkali—Unstable	Light—Unstable
Water—Insol.	

3. Properties

Appearance—white powder
MW—314.5
MP—α = 128°C
    β = 121°C
Crystal Form
    α-Orthorhombic prisms
    β-Orthorhombic needles
Salts, Esters-Acetate,
    caproate
Important Groups for Activity
    —C(3)=O,
    —C(4)=C(5)—
    —C(20)—CH$_3$
       ‖
       O

Solubility
    H_2O—Insol.
    Acet., Alc.—Sol.
    Benz., Chl., Eth.—Sol.
Absn. Max.—240 mμ
Chemical Nature
    Ketone, steroid
α_D = 172-182 (dioxane)

4. Commercial Production

Synthesis from cholesterol, stigmasterol, or diosgenin
Isolation from sow ovary corpora lutea

5. Isolation

Sources—Sow ovary corpora lutea

Methods

    Extract with alkali

    Extract with ether or ether-ethanol (1:3) or methyl acetate-benzene

    Partition between hexane (or petroleum ether) and 70% methyl alcohol

    Purify by chromatography: celite column, thin layer, paper or counter current distribution

6. Determination

Bioassay

    Decidual responses

    Change of progesterone in endometrium

Physicochemical

    Absorption at 240 mμ or at 290 mμ in H_2SO_4

    Yellow fluorescence with $SbCl_3$

    Blue absorption with phosphomolybdic acid

    Protein-binding assay

MEDICAL AND BIOLOGICAL ROLE

1. Species Occurrence, Specificity, Antigenicity

    Occurrence—Found in plants, all vertebrates

    Specificity—Activity crosses species lines

    Antigenicity—No antigenicity reported

2. Units: μg or mg; rabbit unit = 0.6 mg progesterone

3. Normal Blood Levels

    Normal males—0.03 μg/100 ml plasma

    Normal females—0.1-0.3 μg/100 ml plasma

    Pregnant females—10-28 μg/100 ml plasma

4. Administration

    Injection—Intramuscular

    Topical—Not reported

    Oral—As caproate or acetate of 17α-hydroxyprogesterone; various synthetic progestogens used in contraceptive pills in combination with small amounts of estrogens

5. Factors Affecting Release

Inhibitors

    Psychic phenomena

Uterine factor
Feedback mechanisms via hypothalamus
Environmental factors
Stimulators
Hypothalamic agent—LRH (human)—via pituitary and LH
Males—Continuous secretion (low levels)
Females—Continuous secretion in nonspontaneous ovulators (rabbit, ferret, cat); rhythmic in spontaneous ovulators (dog, human)
Psychic and environmental controls
Prolactin or LH, depending on species

6. **Deficiency Symptoms (Humans)**
Termination of pregnancy
Decreased production of steroids
Decreased ovulation
Loss of normal cyclic changes
Decreased development for implantation and gestation

7. **Effects of Overdose, Excess**
Progestational changes
Pregnancy prolongation
Inhibition of uterine growth
Increased Na and K excretion

METABOLIC ROLE

1. **Biosynthesis:** Acetate → Mevalonate → Squalene → Cholesterol → Pregnenolone → Progesterone
Cell Site: Microsomes

2. **Production Sites**
Ovary (follicles, corpus luteum)
Testicles (interstitial cells)
Adrenal cortex (reticularis fasciculata)
Placenta (syncytical trophoblast)

3. **Storage Sites**
Corpora lutea
Adrenal cortex

4. Blood Carriers: Plasma lipoproteins—albumin, transcortin

5. Half-life: About 5 min

6. Target Tissues: Uterus, vagina, cervix, pubic symphysis, ovary, hypothalamus, mammary gland, female sex accessory organs, kidney, adrenal cortex, adenohypophysis

7. Reactions: Reactive form—Unknown

Organ	Enzyme System	Effect
Uterus	Acid phosphatase	Activated
	Carbonic anhydrase	Activated

8. Mode of Action
Cellular
Anabolic: Increases glycoprotein (uterus). Increases glycogen (uterus)
Catabolic: Increases protein catabolism. Increases galactose oxidation
Other: Increases membrane potential. Immediate precursor for other sex hormones. Thermogenic action
Organismal
Increases kidney filtration rate (glomerulus)
Promotes development and growth of uterus and mammary gland
Promotes ovulation and development of sex accessories (female)
Promotes excitation of uterus
Inhibits release of LH

9. Catabolism
Intermediates—Pregnanediol, 17α-hydroxyprogesterone
Excretion products
Urine—Mainly as glucuronates of pregnanediol, pregnanetriol
Feces—Androgens (cow, rat)

MISCELLANEOUS

1. Relationship to Vitamins
Niacin—DPN involved in progesterone synthesis
Vitamin C—Depleted from adrenal cortex or ovary on progesterone formation

2. Relationship to Other Hormones
Estradiol—Antagonist or synergist to progesterone, depending on concentration; made from progesterone

Prolactin, LH—Stimulant for production of progesterone, depending on species

Testosterone—Antagonist or synergist to progesterone, depending on concentration; made from progesterone

Cortisol, Aldosterone—Made from progesterone

STH, T4—Synergist in growth aspects of progesterone

ACTH—Releaser of steroids from adrenal cortex; stimulator of progesterone production

FSH—Synergist with LH in production of progesterone

Relaxin, Oxytocin—Synergist with progesterone in parturition

LRH—Hypothalamic agent stimulating release of LH

3. Unusual Features

Concentration dependence of effects

Primitive type of hormone

Causes maternal behavior in rabbit

Causes pseudopregnancy in nonspontaneous ovulators

Inhibits estrogenic tumors

Anesthetic effects

Androgenic or antiandrogenic, depending on species

Cyclic release in certain species but not in others

4. Possible Relationships of Deficiency Symptoms to Metabolic Action

Loss of pregnancy—Lack of growth and developmental stimulus to uterus by progesterone

Decreased steroid production—Serves as precursor to all other steroid hormones

Decreased ovulation—No progesterone stimulus for development of follicle in ovary

Loss of normal cyclic changes—Feedback mechanisms of progesterone on hypothalamus not controlling (?)

Decreased development for implantation and gestation—Loss of growth and development stimulating action on uterus due to lack of progesterone

35
Testosterone

GENERAL INFORMATION

1. Synonyms: 17β-Hydroxy-4-androsten-3-one, Δ^4-androsten-17β-ol-3-one

2. History

1849—Berthold demonstrated effects of castration prevented by testis transplants

1889—Brown-Sequard claimed rejuvenative powers of testicular extracts

1911—Pezard showed comb growth in capons by injection of testicular extracts

1927—McGee found extracts of bull testis highly potent for male sex hormone activity

1931—Butenandt isolated androsterone from human urine

1935—Laqueur crystallized testosterone from testicular extracts

1935—Butenandt, Ruzicka determined structure and synthesized testosterone

3. Physiological Forms: Androstenedione, testosterone, 11β-hydroxyandrostenedione, adrenosterone

4. Active Analogs and Related Compounds (Androgens)

Natural

11-Hydroxyandrosterone, adrenosterone, 7-hydroxyprogesterone

11-Keto-androsterone

11β-Hydroxyandrostenedione

Synthetic
Ethynyl testosterone, methyltestosterone
6α-chlorotestosterone,   19-nortestosterone,   17α-ethyl-19-nortesto-
sterone

5. **Inactive Analogs and Related Compounds (for Androgenic Activity)**
Cortisone, cortisol, 17-hydroxyprogesterone, lumiandrosterone
17α-hydroxy-11-desoxycorticosterone,   17β-methyl   epitestosterone,
etiocholanolone

6. **Antagonists:**   Estrogens, (except in low concentrations), progesterone,
norethandrolone, 11α-hydroxyprogesterone, methylcholanthrene,
A-norprogesterone

7. **Synergists:**   STH, insulin, other androgens, estrogens (in low concentrations)

8. **Physiological Functions**
Controls secondary male sex characteristics
Maintains functional competence of male reproductive ducts and glands
Increases protein anabolism; maintains spermatogenesis; inhibits gona-
dotrophin
Increases male sex behavior; increases closure of epiphyseal plates

9. **Deficiency Diseases, Disorders**
Male hypogonadism, eunuchoidism
Feminizing testes, hyperplasias of adrenals and testes

10. **Essentiality for Life**
Not essential for life of the organism, but essential for reproduction in all
(male) vertebrates

CHEMISTRY

1. **Structure**

Testosterone, $C_{19}H_{28}O_2$

2. Reactions

Heat—Stable

Acid—Esterifies

Alkali—Fluoresces (conc.)

Water—Insol.

Oxidation—Oxidizes to androstenedione

Reduction—Unstable

Light—Stable

3. Properties

Appearance—White powder

MW—288.4

MP—155°C

Crystal Form—Needles

Salts, Esters

   Propionate, acetate,

   Butyrate, palmitate,

   Stearate, Benzoate

Important Groups for Activity

   $-C(3)=O,-C(17)-OH$

   $-C(4)=C(5)$

Solubility

   H_2O—Insol.

   Acet., Alc.—Sol.

   Benz., Chl., Eth.—Sol.

Absn. Max.—238 mμ

Chemical Nature

   Alcoholic ketone, steroid

$\alpha_D^{24} = 109°$

4. Commercial Production

Microbiological conversion of dehydroandrosterone

Synthesis from cholesterol

5. Isolation

Sources—Urine, blood

Method: Urine

   Hydrolyze with H_2SO_4, extract with organic solvents

   Precipitate with digitonin or Girard's reagent T

   Chromatography: $MgSiO_4$ column or paper or gas

Method: Blood

   Complex with methyl green; transesterify with acetic acid

   Chromatography on Florisil alumina columns

6. Determination

Bioassay

   Growth of capon comb

   Increase in various muscles

   Increase in weight of prostate

   Increase in fructose, citric acid in semen

   Maintenance of spermatogenesis in hypophysectomized rat

Physicochemical—Zimmerman   reaction-(17-oxosteroids);   Pettenkofer

   reaction

MEDICAL AND BIOLOGICAL ROLE

1. **Species Occurrence, Specificity, and Antigenicity**

    Occurrence—Vertebrates (cyclostomes and higher forms), variable types
      of androgens

    Specificity—Variable

      Mammals and Birds—testosterone and androsterone active; pregnen-
        olone inactive

      Rat—pregnenolone active (not in mammals or birds)

    Antigenicity—None reported

2. **Units:**   0.015 mg = I.U.

3. **Normal Blood Levels (Man)**

    Males av. 0.60 μg/100 ml plasma—Androsterone and dehydroepiandro-
      sterone; females av. 0.05 μg/100 ml plasma

4. **Administration**

    Injection—Intramuscular preferred

    Topical—Some cutaneous absorption

    Oral—Active, but less than injected or implanted hormones. More active
      as esters or synthetic androgens

5. **Factors Affecting Release**

    Inhibitors

      Cortisol

      Psychic effects

      Androgens

      Feedback to hypothalamus

    Stimulators

      Photoperiodicity

      Temperature increase, within limits

      Melatonin

      FSH, ACTH, LH, LRH

      Increased blood flow to testis

      Decreased blood levels of androgens or estrogens

6. **Deficiency Symptoms (Humans)**

    Involution of accessory organs (prostate, seminal vesicles)

    Decreased male behavior patterns and libido

    Decreased secondary sex traits

    Poor muscle development and function

Delayed closure of epiphyses
Decreased excretion of 17-keto-steroids in urine

7. Effects of Overdose, Excess: LD_{100} = 325 mg/kg in female rats
Increases libido
Virilization, acne
Increases fat catabolism
Increases androgen and estrogen excretion (17-keto-steroids)
Precocious sex development
Hypertrophy of accessory sex organs
Increases skeletal growth until epiphyses close
Increases muscle mass, hirsutism
Decreases scalp hair growth (?)
Decreases weight—chick, rat

METABOLIC ROLE

1. Biosynthesis: Acetate → Mevalonate → Squalene → Cholesterol
→ Pregnenolone → Progesterone → 17α-hydroxyprogesterone
→ Androstenedione → Testosterone
Cell Sites: Leydig cells in interstitial cells of testis: Agranular cytoplasm

2. Production Sites
Interstitial cells of ovary and testis: Agranular cytoplasm
Adrenal cortex (reticularis fasciculata), embryonic placenta

3. Storage Areas: No data

4. Blood Carriers: Albumin, and a specific β-globulin

5. Half-life: About 4 min

6. Target Tissues
Systemic, fat deposits, muscles, hypothalamus, kidney
Male sex organs, adenohypophysis, hair follicles
Epiphyses of long bones, vocal cords

7. Reactions: Reactive forms
Redox couples—Testosterone ⇌ androstenedione ⇌ androsterone

Organ	Enzyme System	Effect
Kidney	β-Glucuronidase	Activated
	d-Aminooxidase	Activated
	Arginase	Activated
	Alkaline phosphatase	Inhibited
Prostate	Succinic dehydrogenase	Activated
Seminal vesicle	Amino acid activating enzymes	Activated

8. Mode of Action

Cellular

Anabolic—Increases incorporation of amino acids and protein synthesis in muscles, liver, kidney

Catabolic—Increases fat catabolism. Decreases amino acid catabolism

Other

Redox couple regulation of oxidation

Increased mitosis in certain tissues

Increases creatine storage

Membrane effects

Organismal

Increases development of male secondary sex organs and characteristics

Increases growth of muscles, liver, kidney

Androgenic, increases libido

Effects on CNS, male behavior

Increases folliculoid and luteoid activity in immature females

Increases basal metabolism

Maintains positive balances of N, K, Ca, P

Decreases creatinuria

Promotes closure of bone epiphyses

Stimulates red cell production

9. Catabolism

Intermediates—Androstanolone, androstanedione

Excretion Products—Androsterone, etiocholanolone, 17-keto-steroids, dehydroepiandrosterone. In urine, bile, feces-free or conjugated with sulfate or glucuronide. Enterohepatic circulation

MISCELLANEOUS

1. Relationship to Vitamins

Vitamins A, E, C, Folic Acid—Synergists with testosterone for maturation of germ cells and increased anabolic activity

Vitamin B Complex—Male accessory gland maintenance in rat (involution on vit. B deficiency, similar to castration); synergistic in increased metabolic rate

Vitamin D—Synergist with testosterone in bone metabolism

2. Relationship to Other Hormones

Estradiol—Formed from testosterone

LH, LRH, FSH—Stimulators of testosterone formation or release

Estradiol, STH, Insulin—Synergists for action of testosterone (in proper concentrations)

ACTH—stimulates formation of adrenal androgens

Progesterone, Estrogens—Antagonists to testosterone (in proper concentrations)

Cortisol, Estrogens, Androgens—Act as release inhibitors in high concentrations

3. Unusual Features

Multiple sources of production

Fetal sex determination to male via hypothalamus by testosterone

Sensitivity of capon comb to testosterone

Insensitivity of certain muscles to testosterone

Female birds produce testosterone in ovary

Immediate precursor in estrogen synthesis

Two major synthetic routes, three minor ones in adrenals and testes

Social functions in seals affected by androgens

Species differences in effects of testosterone on sperm maturation rate

Dietary effect—Vitamin B deficiency or protein deficiency similar to castration

4. Possible Relationships of Deficiency Symptoms to Metabolic Action

Involution of male accessory organs, decreased secondary sex traits—withdrawal of anabolic effect of testosterone

Decreased male behavior and libido—decreased effect on CNS

Poor muscle development and function—withdrawal of anabolic effect of testosterone

Delayed closure of epiphyses—withdrawal of anabolic effect of testosterone

Decreased excretion of 17-keto-steroids in urine—decreased production of androgens

36
Relaxin

GENERAL INFORMATION

1. **Synonyms:** Releasin, Cervilaxin

2. **History**

    1926—Hisaw cited evidence for a pregnancy hormone which causes relaxation of pelvic ligaments in preparation for parturition

    1930—Fevold *et al.* extracted relaxin from corpora lutea

    1942—Abramowitz isolated relaxin from pregnant rabbit serum

    1955—Lehrman *et al.* isolated and purified relaxin from ovaries of pregnant sows

    1966—Struck and Bhargava isolated first homogeneous preparations of relaxin

3. **Physiological Forms:** *l*-relaxin

4. **Active Analogs and Related Compounds:** Four similar peptides in relaxin family

5. **Inactive Analogs and Related Compounds:** Oxidized or reduced forms of relaxin

6. **Antagonists:** Androgens, corticosterone, high levels of estradiol and progesterone

7. **Synergists:** Low levels of estradiol and progesterone, oxytocin, T4

8. **Physiological Functions**

   Enlargement of birth canal in preparation for parturition

   Separation of symphysis pubis, loss of rigidity in pelvic bones

   Decreases uterine motility

   Maintenance of pregnancy (progesterone + estrogen sparing)

   Increases sensitivity to oxytocin

   Releases oxytocin

   Stimulates mammary gland

   Stimulates imbibition of water in uterus

   Inhibits uterine contraction

9. **Deficiency Diseases, Disorders:**   None known

10. **Essentiality for Life:**   Not essential for human female reproduction, but is essential for other mammalian reproduction. Otherwise not essential for life

CHEMISTRY

1. **Structure:**   Polypeptide (4 peptides with activity have been isolated). Contains Ala, Asp, Cys, Glu, Gly, His, Lys, Ser, Tyr, Val, Arg, guanidine. About 30-40 amino acids in each peptide

2. **Reactions**

   Heat—Stable to 100°C neut. soln.

   Acid—Inactivates (in acidic methanol)

   Alkali—Inactivates (in hot alkali)

   Water—Sol. (acidic)

   Oxidation—Inactivates

   Reduction—Inactivates (SH agents)

   Light—No data

   Proteolytic enzymes—Inactivate

3. **Properties**

   Appearance—Amorphous powder

   MW—4000-5000

   MP—No data

   Crystal Form—Amorphous

   Salts—No data

   Important Groups for Activity

      Guanidine   S—S

                Cys

   Solubility

     H_2O—Sl. sol.

     Acet., Alc.—Insol.

     Benz., Chl., Eth.—Insol.

     Absn. Max.—277.5 mμ

     Chemical Activity—Acidic polypeptide

     Misc.—pI = 4.4

4. **Commercial Production**
    Isolation from pregnant sow ovaries

5. **Isolation**
    Source—Pregnant sow ovaries
    Method—Extraction with trichloroacetic acid, glacial acetic acid, acid-
        acetone; chromatography on columns of DEAE cellulose, IRC-50;
        gel filtration on sephadex G-50

6. **Determination of potency and concentration**
    Bioassay—Measure length of interpubic ligament in mice
        X-Ray photography of innominate bones in estrogen primed guinea
        pig
    Inhibition of motility of mouse uterine segments in vitro
    Physico-chemical—None

MEDICAL AND BIOLOGICAL ROLE

1. **Species Occurrence, Specificity, and Antigenicity**
    Occurrence—Found in mammals, birds, sharks. Relaxin-like substances
        have been isolated from elasmobranch ovaries and bird testes
    Specificity—High; species differences pronounced
    Antigenicity—Moderate; can be antigenic

2. **Units:**   Guinea pig units. Minimal amount necessary to cause appreciable
    separation of symphysis in guinea pig

3. **Normal Blood Levels:**   200 GPU/100 ml (pregnant sow)

4. **Administration**
    Injection—Usually used
    Topical—Not active
    Oral—Not active

5. **Factors Affecting Release**
    Inhibitors
        Androgens
        Corticosterone
        High progesterone level
        High estradiol level

Stimulators
   Low estradiol level
   Low progesterone level
   Pregnenolone

6. **Deficiency Symptoms:** Humans—Unknown

7. **Effects of Overdose, Excess:** Unknown.

METABOLIC ROLE

1. **Biosynthesis**
   Precursors
      11 of 20 standard amino acids, progesterone (cofactor)
      Reducing sugars
      Missing: Try, Asn, Gln, Met, Leu, Ile, Phe, Thr, Pro
   Intermediates—Unknown
   Site(s) in Cell—Unknown

2. **Production Sites:** Corpus luteum in pregnancy. Possibly placenta, uterus
      in some species

3. **Storage Areas:** None

4. **Blood Carriers:** Unknown

5. **Half-life:** Approx. 1 hr

6. **Target Tissues**
   Connective tissue of pubic symphysis
   Uterus (diminution of contractions and softening of cervix)
   Mammary gland
   Vagina

7. **Reactions:** Reactive Forms: Unknown

Organ	Enzyme System	Effect
Pubic symphysis	Collagen depolymerases	Activated
Liver	Cholesterol biosynthesis	Inhibited
Uterus	Alkaline phosphatase	Increased

8. Mode of Action
Cellular
    Anabolic—Increases uterine glycogen synthesis
    Catabolic—No data
  Other—Decreases membrane potential of myometrium. Enzyme activator
Organismal
    Increases vascularity of pubic symphysis
    Imbibition of water; disaggregation and depolymerization of muco-
      proteins in ground structure of symphysis
    Increases glycogen and water content of uterus, also dry weight and
      N content
    Decreases uterine motility
    Softens cervix of uterus
    Increases uterine sensitivity to oxytocin
    Stimulates release of oxytocin
    Relaxes interpubic ligament

9. Catabolism
Intermediates—Peptides, amino acids
Excretion products—Ammonia, CO_2, H_2O, amino acids, 1-4% relaxin in
  urine

MISCELLANEOUS

1. **Relationship to Vitamins:** Vitamin C—Maintains mucoprotein ground
substance in connective tissue, affected by relaxin

2. **Relationship to Other Hormones**
  Estradiol—Relaxin works in conjunction with estrogens—synergistic or
    antagonistic depending on concentration (requires estrogen
    "priming")
  Oxytocin—Relaxin may initiate oxytocin release
  STH—Relaxin may require growth hormone for relaxation of interpubic
    ligament
  Progesterone—Synergistic or antagonistic depending on concentration
  TSH—Increased biosynthesis of TSH stimulated by relaxin
  Testosterone, Corticosterone—Act as release inhibitors

3. **Unusual Features**
  Hormone of pregnancy only
  Strictly female hormone, although general effects noted in body

Found in rooster testes—No known function
Inhibits cholesterol biosynthesis, hypocholesteremic
Increases hydrolysis of collagen

4. Possible Relationships of Deficiency Symptoms to Metabolic Action:
Unknown

37
Epinephrine

GENERAL INFORMATION

1. **Synonyms:** Adrenaline, Adrenin, Suprarenin, Vasotonin, Vasocon-strictine, Adrenamine, Levorenine

2. **History**

   1895—Oliver and Shafer demonstrated pressor effect of suprarenal extracts

   1899—Abel named pressor agent epinephrine

   1901—Takamine, Aldrich isolated epinephrine from animal adrenal glands

   1904—Stolz
   1905—Dakin } synthesized *dl*-epinephrine

   1908—Flacher responsible for resolution of *dl*-form of epinephrine

   1910—Barger and Dale defined sympathomimetic amines and their properties

   1958—Pratesi determined configuration of epinephrine

3. **Physiological Forms:** *l*-Epinephrine

4. **Active Analogs and Related Compounds**

   d-epinephrine (1/15 as active as *l*-isomers), norepinephrine, dopamine, ephedrin, benzedrine, paredrine, tyramine, isoproterenol

5. **Inactive Analogs and Related Compounds:** DOPA

6. **Antagonists:**   Insulin, ergotamine, dibenamine, oxytocin, dibenzyline, tetraethylammonium chloride

7. **Synergists:**   Glucagon, T4, cortisol, ACTH

8. **Physiological Functions**

Blood Circulation—Increases blood pressure (pressor agent), peripheral vasodilator, increases heart output and rate, flow increase in brain, liver, and skeletal muscle

Kidney—Reduces glomerular filtration rate

Lung, intestine, genital system—Inhibited motility

Metabolic effects—Increases O_2 consumption, increases temperature, increases BMR, increases gluconeogenesis

CNS effects—Restlessness, anxiety

Pituitary effects—Stimulates production and release of ACTH and corticoids

Emergency hormone—Stress reactions

9. **Deficiency Diseases, Disorders:**   Pheochromocytoma (chromaffin cells)

10. **Essentiality for Life:**   Not absolutely essential for life of organism; possible shortening of life span due to decreased response to emergencies

CHEMISTRY

1. **Structure**

l-Epinephrine, $C_9H_{13}NO_3$

2. **Reactions**

Heat—Decomposes at 215°C
Acid—Inactivates
Alkali—Unstable—Very sol. in dil. NaOH. Insol. in NH_4OH
Water—Sol., basic

Oxidation—Oxidizes easily
Reduction—Stable
Light—Fluorescent in UV; darkens on exposure, forms adreno-chrome

3. **Properties**

Appearance—white crystalline powder

MW—183.2

MP—211-212°C

Crystal Form—No data

Salts—HCl

Important Groups for Activity

Phenol, amine, alcohol

$-C(4)OH$, $-NH-$, $-CHOH$

Solubility

H_2O—Sparingly

Acet., Alc.—Insol.

Benz., Chl., Eth.—Insol.

Absn. Max.—279 mμ

Chemical Nature

Catecholamine

Secondary amine

$\alpha_D^{25} = -53.5°$ (0.5 N HCl)

4. **Commercial Production**

Adrenal gland extractions

Synthetic production

5. **Isolation**

Sources—Adrenal medulla, urine, blood

Methods

Hydrolysis of conjugates, if any, boiling at pH 2, 20 min

Extraction with acidic ethanol or n-butanol

Purification via paper chromatography

6. **Determination**

Bioassay

Inhibition of movement of isolated rat uterus

Constrictor action on artery of denervated rabbit ear

Physicochemical

Iodochrome oxidation to distinguish norepinephrine from epinephrine

Fluorescence in alkali

Color reaction with ferric chloride

MEDICAL AND BIOLOGICAL ROLE

1. **Species Occurrence, Specificity, and Antigenicity**

Occurrence—Found in all vertebrates and some invertebrates

Specificity—None, full interspecific potency

Antigenicity—None

2. **Units:** None; by weight

3. **Normal Blood Levels (Man):** Approximately 0.01 μg/100 ml plasma (venous)

4. **Administration**
    Injection—Subcutaneous, intramuscular
    Topical—Active (electrophoretic application)
    Oral—Possible, but slow

5. **Factors Affecting Release**
    Inhibitors—Nerve controls, excess catecholamines
    Stimulators—Nicotine, histamine, reserpine, acetylcholine, morphine,
        ether, ACTH, glucocorticoids, low blood sugar, stress, insulin,
        psychic (hypothalamus) nerve controls, trauma, exercise

6. **Deficiency Symptoms** Not fatal, but organism cannot respond to emer-
        gency, hard work, temperature extreme, emotional disturbance

7. **Effects of Overdose, Excess**
    Decreases oxygen consumption, BMR, clotting time,
    Tachycardia, restlessness, anxiety, fatigue, inhibited G.I. tract,
    Increases heart rate, respiration, pallor, blood sugar, sweat, blood flow
        (muscle)
    Ventricular fibrillation, paroxystic or sustained hypertension

METABOLIC ROLE

1. **Biosynthesis:**   Phenylalanine → Tyrosine → 3,4-Dihydroxyphenylalanine
    (DOPA) → 3,4-Dihydroxyphenylethylamine (Dopamine) → Nore-
    pinephrine → Epinephrine
    Site(s) in cell: In golgi (osmiophilic granules)

2. **Production Sites:**   Chromaffin cells in gut and adrenal medulla

3. **Storage Areas:**   Chromaffin cells in liver and gut

4. **Blood Carriers:**   Free in blood or conjugated with sulfate or glucuronides,
        or combined with albumin

5. **Half-life:**   About 2 min

6. **Target Tissues:**   Systemic, vascular system, liver, muscles

7. **Reactions**
    Reactive intermediate—Cyclic AMP—(secondary messenger)

Organ	Enzyme System	Effect
Muscle and liver	Phosphorylase b	Activated
	Adenyl cyclase	Activated
	Phosphorylase b kinase	Activated
	Synthetase I kinase	Activated
	Synthetase I	Inhibited
Adipose tissue	Lipase	Activated
	Adenyl cyclase	Activated

8. Mode of Action
Cellular

Anabolic—No data

Catabolic —Increases glycogenolysis in liver, increases fat catabolism

Other

Decreases glucose entry into cells of skeletal muscle

Increases glucose entry into heart, brain and adipose tissue cells

Increases cyclic AMP

Supresses mitosis

Calorigenic action

Organismal

Increases—Systolic pressure; blood flow to skeletal muscles, liver; blood sugar; lipolysis; blood K^+; O_2 consumption (BMR), glucose absorption from gut, mental alertness, sweating

Decreases—Glucose tolerance, eosinophils, blood flow to capillaries of skin and kidney, plasma volume

Lightens chromatophores

9. Catabolism
Intermediates—3,4-dihydroxymandelic acid

Excretion Products—Free (0.5 to 2%) or as metanephrine (3-methoxy, 4OH-mandelic acid)

MISCELLANEOUS

1. **Relationship to Vitamins:**   Vitamin C—Maintains reduced state of epinephrine. Vitamins C, B_6, B_{12}, folic acid—Cofactors in synthesis of epinephrine from phenylalanine

2. **Relationship to Other Hormones**

Norepinephrine—Immediate precursor to epinephrine

Insulin—Antagonist to epinephrine

Glucagon, T4, ACH—Synergists to epinephrine

TSH—Released by epinephrine
Prolactin—Blocking of milk ejection by epinephrine
Cortisol, Cortisone—Synergistic in stress response
Oxytocin—Epinephrine antagonistic in milk ejection

3. **Unusual Features**

Active at 1.4 parts per billion
Absent in developing fetus; Proportion of NOR/EP = 1:4 in adult human adrenal (reverse in chick); blocks milk ejection; rabbit most sensitive; behavioral effects
Proportion of NOR/EP varies in invertebrates
Increases mental alertness
Calorigenic action

4. **Possible Relationships of Deficiency Symptoms to Metabolic Action**

Decreased emergency response—Decreased lipolysis in adipose tissue results in decreased glucose energy (ATP) available for stress reaction
Decreased response to emotional disturbances, temperature extremes, hard work—as in the previous symptom

38
Norepinephrine

GENERAL INFORMATION

1. **Synonyms:** Noradrenaline, arterenol, levarterenol

2. **History**

   1898—Lewandowsky ⎱ Noted similarity of effects of adrenal gland
   1901—Langley ⎰ extracts and stimulation of sympathetic nerves, on tissues

   1904—Eliot proposed sympathetic nerve endings release epinephrine-like substance
   1910—Barger and Dale synthesized norepinephrine
   1927—Cannon and Uridil noted that liver releases epinephrine-like substance called sympathin on stimulation of sympathetic nerves
   1948—Tullar resolved *dl*-form of norepinephrine
   1951—Euler demonstrated sympathin to be norepinephrine
   1959—Pratesi established configuration of norepinephrine

3. **Physiological Forms:** *l*-Norepinephrine

4. **Active Analogs and Related Compounds:** Dopamine, ephedrine, *d*-norepinephrine, *d*-epinephrine (1/15 as active as *l*-isomers)

5. **Inactive Analogs and Related Compounds:** DOPA

6. **Antagonists:** Insulin, vasopressin

248

7. **Synergists:**   Epinephrine, serotonin, cortisol, cortisone, glucagon

8. **Physiological Functions**
   Blood circulation—Increases blood pressure, peripheral vasoconstrictor, without change or slight decrease in output and heart rate. No flow increase in brain, liver, or muscle
   Kidney—Decreases glomerular filtration rate
   Lung, intestine, genital system—Inhibited
   Metabolic effects—Weak epinephrine effect.
   CNS effects—Adrenergic transmitter agent at synapses, no brain excitation
   Pituitary effects—None
   Maintenance hormone—Diurnal regulation
   Immediate precursor of epinephrine

9. **Deficiency Diseases, Disorders**
   Neuroblastoma
   Pheochromocytoma

10. **Essentiality for Life:**   Not absolutely essential for life of organism, except if other neurotransmitters not available

CHEMISTRY

1. **Structure**

   l-Norepinephrine, $C_8H_{11}NO_3$

2. **Reactions**

   Heat—Unstable
   Acid—Inactivates
   Alkali—Very sol. dil. NaOH; Insol. NH_4OH
   Water—Soluble, alkaline

   Oxidation—Easily oxidizes to noradrenochrome
   Reduction—Stable
   Light—No fluorescence in UV

3. **Properties**

   Appearance—Colorless crystals
   MW—169.2
   MP—145-146°C
   Crystal Form—No data

   Salts—HCl
   Important Groups for Activity
   Alcohol—CHOH, phenol, —C(4)OH, amine, ($-NH_2$)

Solubility
  H_2O sparingly
  Acet., Alc.—Sl. sol.
  Benz., Chl., Eth.—Sl. sol.
Absn. Max.—279 mμ

Chemical Nature—Catecholamine; primary amine
$\alpha_D^{25} = -37.3$ (HCl)
Misc.—pK = 8.8, 9.98

4. **Commercial Production:** Synthetic production

5. **Isolation**
  Sources—Adrenal medulla, blood, urine
  Methods
    Hydrolysis of conjugates, if any—Boil at pH 2, 20 min
    Extraction with acidic ethanol or n-butanol

6. **Determination**
  Bioassay—Pressor effect in cat, rat
  Physicochemical
    Colorimetric—Ferric chloride complex
    Fluorometric—Condense with ethylenediamine

MEDICAL AND BIOLOGICAL ROLE

1. **Species, Occurrence, Specificity, and Antigenicity**
  Occurrence—Found in all vertebrates and some invertebrates
  Specificity—None; full, interspecific potency
  Antigenicity—None

2. **Units:** None; by weight

3. **Normal Blood Levels (Man):** Approx. 0.05 μg/100 ml plasma (venous)

4. **Administration**
  Injection—Usual
  Topical—By electrophoresis through skin
  Oral—Inactive

5. **Factors Affecting Release**
  Inhibitors—Nerve controls, excess catecholamines
  Stimulators—ACH, nicotine, histamine, Tyr, Phe, low blood sugar, low
    T4, nerve controls, stress, trauma, reserpine, morphine

6. **Deficiency Symptoms**
   Poor nerve condition
   Orthostatic hypotension—Fainting on standing up, dizziness, light-headedness

7. **Effects of Overdose, Excess:**   Bradycardia, pheochromocytoma

METABOLIC ROLE

1. **Biosynthesis:**   Phenylalanine → Tyrosine → 3,4-Dihydroxyphenylalanine (DOPA) → 3,4-Dihydroxyphenylethylamine (Dopamine) — Norepinephrine
   Site(s) in cell—Osmiophilic granules in golgi apparatus

2. **Production Sites**
   Adrenal medulla
   Adrenergic nerve endings
   Chromaffin cells—sympathetic nerves and ganglia, gut

3. **Storage Areas:**   Chromaffin cells in liver and gut, intraaxonal spaces, adrenal medulla

4. **Blood Carriers:**   Free or sulfate, glucuronide esters

5. **Half-life:**   2 min or less

6. **Target Tissues:**   Systemic, esp. vascular system, lung, eye

7. **Reactions:**   Reactive intermediate: Cyclic AMP—secondary messenger

Organ	Enzyme Systems	Effect
Muscle and liver	Adenyl cyclase	Activated
	Phosphorylase b	Activated
	Phosphorylase b kinase	Activated
	Synthetase I kinase	Activated
	Synthetase I	Inhibited
Adipose tissue	Adenyl cyclase	Activated
	Lipase	Activated

8. **Mode of Action**
   Cellular
      Anabolic—No data

Catabolic
  Increased CHO catabolism
  Increased glycogen to glucose conversion
  Increased fat catabolism
Other—No data
Organismal
  Decreases—Pulse, blood flow, G.I. and genital activity, respiration
  Increases—Diastolic and systolic pressure, vasodilation of coronary
    arteries, lipid mobilization, glucose absorption from gut
  Bradycardia
  Vasoconstrictor

9. **Catabolism**
    Intermediates—3,4-dihydroxymandelic acid
    Excretion products—Free in urine (3-6%), normetanephrine, 3-methoxy,
      4-hydroxymandelic acid

MISCELLANEOUS

1. **Relationship to Vitamins:**   Vitamin C protects against oxidation of
    norepinephrine. Vitamins B_6, C, folic acid—cofactors in synthesis
    of norepinephrine from phenylalanine

2. **Relationship to Other Hormones**
    Epinephrine—Derivative of norepinephrine; synergist also
    Insulin—Antagonist to norepinephrine, secretion inhibited by norepine-
      phrine
    Serotonin, Cortisol, Cortisone—Synergists to norepinephrine
    T4, ACH—Stimulators for release of norepinephrine

3. **Unusual Features**
    Neurohumor—Much carried intraaxonally
    EP/NOR = 4/1 in medulla (man)
    Diurnal (higher in day)
    No behavioral effects
    Increases pigment concentration in skin
    Main amine in fetus
    Anticipatory type, i.e., normal plasma maintenance

4. **Possible Relationships of Deficiency Symptoms to Metabolic Action**
    Poor nerve conduction—Lack of transmitter agent
    Dizziness, light-headedness, fainting—Low blood pressure

Summarizing
Tables

TABLE 1. Characteristics of Vitamins

(+ = present in structure or function ± = slightly)
(− = catabolic or inhibiting effect)

Structural Component or Function	A	B_1	B_2	B_6	B_{12}	C	D	E	K	Biotin	F.A.[a]	Niacin	P.A.[b]
Amino Acid									+	+	+		+
Purine, pyrimidine (derivative)		+	+		+						+		
Benzene ring			+					+	+		+		
Pyridine ring				+								+	
Isoprene group (derivative)	+						+	+	+				
Sugar (derivative)			+		+	+							
Alcohol groups	+	+	+	+	+	+	+	+			+		+
Double bonds ($-C=C-$)	+	+	+	+	+	+	+	+	+		+	+	
Elements other than CHON		S			Co					S			
Redox agent		+	+	+	+	+		+	+		+	+	
PO_4 complex *in vivo*		+	+	+	+		+				+	+	+
Antioxidant		+		+	+	+		+					
Biosynthesis via Cholesterol pathway	+						+	+	+				

254

Property	1	2	3	4	5	6	7	8	9	10	11	12
Anabolic functions	+	+	+	+	+	+	+	+	+	+	+	+
Catabolic functions	+	±	±	+	+	+	+	+	+	+	+	+
Stored in organism (man)	+	±	±	±	±	±	±	+	+	±	+	±
Available from intestinal bacteria (man)	±	±	±	±				+	+			
Toxic in excess (man)	+	+	+	+		+		±			+	
Mitosis effect				+	−						+	
Mitochondrial sites	+	+	+	+	+	+	+	+	+		+	+
Chloroplast sites	+ᵍ	+				+	+	+			+	
Microsomal sites						+	+				+	
Membrane sites	+	+	+	+	+	+	+		+			
Protein synthesis				+	±		+	+				
Amino acid synthesis		−	−					±	±		−	−
CHO synthesis	+	−	−	+	+	+	+	+	+		−	−

ᵃFolic acid.   ᵇPantothenic acid.   ᵍCarotenoids.

TABLE 1. Characteristics of Vitamins (cont.)

(+ = stimulating effect or present in organelles)

Structural Component or Function	A	B₁	B₂	B₆	B₁₂	C	D	E	K	Biotin	F.A.ᵃ	Niacin	P.A.ᵇ
TCA Cycle effect		+	+									+	+
Lipid synthesis					+								±
Fatty acid synthesis				+						+			±
Nucleic acid synthesis					+								
Purine pyrimidine synthesis					+					+	+		
Mineral metabolism	Ca					Fe, Ca	Ca	Se					+
H₂O metabolism													+
Hormone Synthesis	Prog.ᵉ Cortic.ᶜ Andro.ᵈ	ACHᶠ		ACHᶠ Nor. Serot.		Serot. Gluc.						+	ACHᶠ
Sterol Synthesis	+			+		+						+	+

ᵃFolic acid. ᵇPantothenic acid. ᶜCorticosterone. ᵈAndrostenedione. ᵉProgesterone. ᶠAcetylcholine.

256

TABLE 2. Synergisms (+) and Antagonisms (−) Among the Vitamins

Vitamins	A	B_1	B_2	B_6	B_{12}	C	D	E	K	Biotin	F.A.[a]	Niacin	P.A.[b]
A			+	+	+	±							
B_1			+	+	+							+	+
B_2	+	+		+	+					+	+	+	+
B_6		+	+			+	+	+		+	+		
B_{12}	+	+	+			+	+			+	+	+	+
C	+		+	+			+	+		+			+
D											+		
E			+	+	+	+				+			
K						+	+						
Biotin			+	+	+						+		+
F.A.[a]			+	+	+	+	+	+				+	+
Niacin		+	+	+	+	+					+		+
P.A.[b]		+	+	+	+					+	+	+	

[a] Folic acid.   [b] Pantothenic acid.

TABLE 3. Characteristics of Hormones

Hormones[a]	Amino Acid Units (Proteins, Peptides)	S—S Bonds	CHO Component	Steroid Unit	Catecholamine	Elements Other Than CHON	Redox Couple in Vivo	Mediated Via Cyclic AMP	CHO (Anabolism +, Catabolism −)	Lipid + / Fat − (Anabolism +, Catabolism −)	Protein (Amino Acid) (Anabolism +, Catabolism −)	Nucleic Acid (or Purine, pyrim.) (Anabolism +, Catabolism −)	Steroid (Anabolism +, Catabolism −)	Mineral and H_2O Balance	Mitotic Effect (Increase +, Decrease −)	Membrane Effect	Kidney Function	Blood Pressure	Nerve Function
ACTH	+					S		+	−	−			+[a]						
Aldos.				+			+		±	−	±	±		+		+	+		
Cort.				+			+		±	±	±	±		+	−	+	+		
Epi.				+	+		+	+	−	±	+	+	+[b]	+	−	+	+	+	+
Est.									±	+	+				+	+			+
FSH	+	+	+			S		+	+				+			+			
Gluc.	+	+				S		+	−	−	−			+		+	+		
GH (STH)	+	+				S		+	+	−	+	+		+	+	+	+		
(HRH)	+	+				S		+			+					+			

In.	+	+			S	±	+	+	+	+	+		+	+		+
LH	+	+	+		S	−	+		+	+	+	+		+		+
MSH	+				S	+					+			+		
Norepi.			+		+	−	−		+		+	+	+	+	+	+
Oxy.	+	+			S				+	+	+		+	+	+	+
PTH	+				S	+			+	+	+	+	+		+	
Prog.			+			±	±	±	+	+	+	+	+	+		+
Prol.	+	+			S	+	+	+	+	+	+	+	+	+	+	+
Relax.	+	+			S	±	±		+	+	+	+	+	+		
Test.			+	+		−	−		+	+	+	+	+	+		+
TCT	+	+			S	+	+		+	+	+	+	+	+	+	+
T4	+				−	−	−		+	+	+	+	+	+		+
TSH	+	+			S	+	±		+	+		+		+		+
Vaso.	+	+			S	−	−		+	+	+		+	+	+	+

aSee list of abbreviations for full name. bRelease.

259

TABLE 4. Synergisms (+) and Antagonisms (−)

Hormones[a]	ACTH	Aldos.	Cort.	Epi.	Est.	FSH.	Gluc.	GH (STH)	HRH	In.	LH
ACTH			±	+				±		−	
Aldos.			−		−			+			
Cort.	±	−		+	±		+	±		−	
Epi.	+		+				+			−	
Est.		−	±					+		+	
FSH								+			+
Gluc.			+	+						−	
GH (STH)	±	+	±		+	+				±	
HRH											
In.	−		−	−	+	−	−	±			±
LH					+					±	
MSH			±	−				+			
Norepi.			+	+			+			−	
Oxy.		+	±	−	+			+			
PTH			±		±[b]			−			
Prog.		−	+		±			+			
Prol.			+		±			+			±
Relax.		−			±						
Test.		−			±			+		+	
TCT					+						
T4	±		+	+	+	+		+		−	+
TSH	+							+			
Vaso.			±	−	+			+			

[a] See list of abbreviations for full name.   [b] Birds.

Among the Hormones

Hormones[a]	MSH	Norepi.	Oxy.	PTH	Prog.	Prol.	Relax.	Test.	TCT	T4	TSH	Vaso.
ACTH										±	+	
Aldos.			+	−								±
Cort.	±	+	±	±	+	+	−	−		+		−
Epi.	−	+	−							+		+
Est.			+	±[b]	±	±	±	±	+	+		
FSH										+		
Gluc.		+										
GH (STH)	+		+	−	+	+		+		+	+	+
HRH												
In.		−						+		−		
LH					±					+		
MSH										+	+	
Norepi.												−
Oxy.				±	+	+				+		
PTH						+		−	−	−		
Prog.			±			+	±	±		+		
Prol.			+	+	+			−		+		+
Relax.			+		±			−		+		
Test.				−	±	−	−					+
TCT			−									
T4	+		+	−	+	+	+				+	+
TSH	+									+		
Vaso.		−			+			+		+		

[a]See list of abbreviations for full name.   [b]Birds.

TABLE 5. Synergisms (+) and Antagonisms (−) Between Vitamins and Hormones

Hormones[a]	A	B₁	B₂	B₆	B₁₂	C	D	E	K	Biotin	F.A.[b]	Niacin	P.A.[c]
ACTH	+									+		+	+
Aldos.													
Cort.					±	−							
Epi.				+	+								
Est.	−		−			+	+				+		
FSH													
Gluc.				+									
GH (STH)	+	+	+	+	+	+	+	+	+	+	+	+	+
				All related to growth									
HRH													
In.		+	+		−								
LH						+							
MSH	+												
Norepi.				+	+								
Oxy.													
PTH						±							
Prog.													
Prol.[e]	+	+	+	+	+·	+	+	+	+	+	+	+	+
Relax.													
Test.	+	+	+			+	+	+		+	+		
TCT						−							
T4	±ᵈ	+	+	−		+		−				+	
TSH	−ᵈ		+										
Vaso.													

[a] See list of abbreviations for full name. [b] Folic acid. [c] Pantothenic acid. [d] Large Doses.
[e] All synergistic when acting as a growth hormone.

TABLE 6. Principal Functional Relationships of Vitamins and Hormones

( ) = indirect effect   ＿＿= Major Effect

Function	Vitamin(s)[a]	Hormone(s)[a]
Bone and Ca metabolism	A, C, <u>D</u>	Cort., (ACTH), Est., GH <u>PTH</u>, Test., <u>TCT</u>, T4, (TSH)
Circulation, blood cells	B_6, B_{12}, C, E, K, Bio., <u>F.A.</u>, P.A.	Cort., (ACTH), <u>Epi.</u>, Norepi., Vaso.
Digestion and absorption	B_1, B_{12}, <u>D</u>, <u>E</u>, <u>F.A.</u>, <u>Nia.</u>	Cort., (ACTH), Gluc., <u>In.</u>, PTH, <u>T4</u> (TSH)
Epithelium, skin (membrane effect)	<u>A</u>, B_2, B_{12}, D, <u>Bio.</u>, P.A.	<u>Aldos.</u>, Cort., (ACTH), Epi., Est., GH, In., Norepi., Oxy., Prog., Relax., Test., T4 (TSH), <u>Vaso.</u>
Fat and CHO metabolism	<u>B_1</u>, <u>B_2</u>, B_6, B_{12}, Bio., Nia., <u>P.A.</u>	(ACTH), Aldos., Cort., Epi., Est., <u>Gluc.</u>, GH, <u>In.</u>, Norepi., T4 (TSH), Test.
Growth	All, by definition	All, by definition; Esp.: <u>Est.</u>, <u>GH</u>, <u>In.</u>, <u>T4</u> (TSH), <u>Test.</u>
Metabolic rate, temperature (TCA Cycle)	<u>B_1</u>, <u>B_2</u>, C, E, K, <u>Nia.</u>, P.A.	<u>Epi.</u>, Norepi., Prog., <u>T4</u>, (TSH), Test.
Nerve function, psyche	A, <u>B_1</u>, B_2, B_{12}, C, Bio., Nia., <u>F.A.</u>, P.A.	Cort., (ACTH), <u>Epi.</u>, Norepi., Prol., Test., <u>T4</u>, (TSH), Est.
Pigmentation	B_6, C, F.A., <u>Nia.</u>	(ACTH), Cort., <u>MSH</u>
Pregnancy, lactation	All required at higher levels	Cort., (ACTH), <u>Est.</u> (FSH), GH, In., (LH), <u>Oxy.</u>, <u>Prol.</u>, <u>Prog.</u>, <u>Relax.</u>, T4, (TSH)
Salt (Na) and H_2O metabolism	B_6, <u>P.A.</u> (A, C, E, Nia.)	<u>Aldos.</u>, Cort., (ACTH), Epi., Gluc., GH., (In.), Norepi., Oxy., Prog., T4, (TSH), <u>Vaso.</u>
Stress, immunity	C, P.A., <u>A</u> (B_1, B_2, B_6, K, Bio., F.A.)	Aldo., <u>Cort.</u>, (ACTH), Est.
Visual mechanisms	<u>A</u>, B_2	

[a] See list of abbreviations for full name.

TABLE 7. Food and Nutrition Board, National Academy of Science— National Research Council Recommended Daily Dietary Allowances,[1] Revised 1968

Designed for the maintenance of good nutrition of practically all healthy people in the U.S.A.

	Age[2] Years From Up to	Weight Kg (lb)		Height cm (in.)		Kcal	Protein g	Fat Soluble Vitamins		
								Vit. A Activity I.U.	Vit. D I.U.	Vit. E Activity I.U.
Infants	0–1/6	4	9	55	22	kg x 120	kg x 2.2[5]	1500	400	5
	1/6–1/2	7	15	63	25	kg x 110	kg x 2.0[5]	1500	400	5
	1/2–1	9	20	72	28	kg x 100	kg x 1.8[5]	1500	400	5
Children	1–2	12	26	81	32	1100	25	2000	400	10
	2–3	14	31	91	36	1250	25	2000	400	10
	3–4	16	35	100	39	1400	30	2500	400	10
	4–6	19	42	110	43	1600	30	2500	400	10
	6–8	23	51	121	48	2000	35	3500	400	15
	8–10	28	62	131	52	2200	40	3500	400	15
Males	10–12	35	77	140	55	2500	45	4500	400	20
	12–14	43	95	151	59	2700	50	5000	400	20
	14–18	59	130	170	67	3000	60	5000	400	25
	18–22	67	147	175	69	2800	60	5000	400	30
	22–35	70	154	175	69	2800	65	5000	–	30
	35–55	70	154	173	68	2600	65	5000	–	30
	55–75+	70	154	171	67	2400	65	5000	–	30
Females	10–12	35	77	142	56	2250	50	4500	400	20
	12–14	44	97	154	61	2300	50	5000	400	20
	14–16	52	114	157	62	2400	55	5000	400	25
	16–18	54	119	160	63	2300	55	5000	400	25
	18–22	58	128	163	64	2000	55	5000	400	25
	22–35	58	128	163	64	2000	55	5000	–	25
	35–55	58	128	160	63	1850	55	5000	–	25
	55–75+	58	128	157	62	1700	55	5000	–	25
Pregnancy						+200	65	6000	400	30
Lactation						+1000	75	8000	400	30

1. The allowance levels are intended to cover individual variations among most normal persons as they live in the United States under usual environmental stresses. The recommended allowances can be attained with a variety of common foods, providing other nutrients for which human requirements have been less well defined. See text [of Recommended Dietary Allowances, National Research Council Pub. #1694] for more detailed discussion of allowances and of nutrients not tabulated.

2. Entries on lines for age range 22–35 years represent the reference man and woman at age 22. All other entries represent allowances for the midpoint of the specified age range.

Water Soluble Vitamins							Minerals				
Ascorbic Acid mg	Folacin[3] mg	Niacin mg. equiv.[4]	Ribo-flavin mg	Thiamine mg	Vit. B_6 mg	Vit. B_{12} µg	Calcium gm	Phos-phorus gm	Iodine µg	Iron mg	Mag-nesium mg
35	0.05	5	0.4	0.2	0.2	1.0	0.4	0.2	25	6	40
35	0.05	7	0.5	0.4	0.3	1.5	0.5	0.4	40	10	60
35	0.1	8	0.6	0.5	0.4	2.0	0.6	0.5	45	15	70
40	0.1	8	0.6	0.6	0.5	2.0	0.7	0.7	55	15	100
40	0.2	8	0.7	0.6	0.6	2.5	0.8	0.8	60	15	150
40	0.2	9	0.8	0.7	0.7	3	0.8	0.8	70	10	200
40	0.2	11	0.9	0.8	0.9	4	0.8	0.8	80	10	200
40	0.2	13	1.1	1.0	1.0	4	0.9	0.9	100	10	250
40	0.3	15	1.2	1.1	1.2	5	1.0	1.0	110	10	250
40	0.4	17	1.3	1.3	1.4	5	1.2	1.2	125	10	300
45	0.4	18	1.4	1.4	1.6	5	1.4	1.4	135	18	350
55	0.4	20	1.5	1.5	1.8	5	1.4	1.4	150	18	400
60	0.4	18	16	1.4	2.0	5	0.8	0.8	140	10	400
60	0.4	18	1.7	1.4	2.0	5	0.8	0.8	140	10	350
60	0.4	17	1.7	1.3	2.0	5	0.8	0.8	125	10	350
60	0.4	14	1.7	1.2	2.0	6	0.8	0.8	110	10	350
40	0.4	15	1.3	1.1	1.4	5	1.2	1.2	110	18	300
45	0.4	15	1.4	1.2	1.6	5	1.3	1.3	115	18	350
50	0.4	16	1.4	1.2	1.8	5	1.3	1.3	120	18	350
50	0.4	15	1.5	1.2	2.0	5	1.3	1.3	115	18	350
50	0.4	15	1.5	1.2	2.0	5	1.3	1.3	115	18	350
55	0.4	13	1.5	1.0	2.0	5	0.8	0.8	100	18	300
55	0.4	13	1.5	1.0	2.0	5	0.8	0.8	90	18	300
55	0.4	13	1.5	1.0	2.0	6	0.8	0.8	80	10	300
60	0.8	15	1.8	+0.1	2.5	8	+0.4	+0.4	125	18	450
60	0.5	20	2.0	+0.5	2.5	6	+0.5	+0.5	150	18	450

3. The folacin allowances refer to dietary sources as determined by Lactobacillus casei assay. Pure forms of folacin may be effective in doses less than 1/4 of the RDA.

4. Niacin equivalents include dietary sources of the vitamin itself plus 1 mg equivalent for each 60 mg of dietary tryptophan.

5. Assumes protein equivalent to human milk. For proteins not 100 percent utilized factors should be increased proportionately.

Table reproduced with permission of the National Academy of Sciences.

Principal
References

PRINCIPAL REFERENCES

General

1. Altman, P. L. and Dittmer, D. S. (Eds.), *Biology Data Book*, Fed. Am. Soc. Exp. Biol., Washington, D.C. (1964).
2. Altman, P. L. and Dittmer, D. S. (Eds.), *Blood and Other Body Fluids*, Fed. Am. Soc. Exp. Biol., Washington, D.C. (1961).
3. Altman, P. L. and Dittmer, D. S. (Eds.), *Growth*, Fed. Am. Soc. Exp. Biol., Washington, D.C. (1962).
4. Altman, P. L. and Dittmer, D. S. (Eds.), *Metabolism*, Fed. Am. Soc. Exp. Biol., Washington, D.C. (1968).
5. Boyer, P. D. and Snell, E. E. (Eds.), *Annual Reviews of Biochemistry*, Vols. 36—39, Annual Reviews, Inc., Palo Alto, Calif. (1967—70).
6. Conn, E. E. and Stumpf, P. K., *Outlines of Biochemistry*, 2nd Ed., Wiley, New York (1966).
7. Dawson, R. M. C., Elliott, D. C., Elliot, W. H., and Jones, K. M. (Eds.), *Data for Biochemical Research*, 2nd Ed., Oxford Univ. Press. New York and Oxford (1969).
8. Diem, K. (Ed.), *Documenta Geigy Scientific Tables,* 6th Ed., Geigy Pharmaceuticals, Ardsley, N.Y. (1962).
9. Goodman, L. S. and Gilman, A. (Ed.), *The Pharmaceutical Basis of Therapeutics*, 4th Ed., Macmillan, New York (1970).
10. Greenberg, D. M. (Ed.), *Metabolic Pathways*, 3rd Ed., Vols. I—IV, Academic Press, New York and London (1967).
11. Harris, R. S., Wool, I. G., and Loraine, J. A. (Eds.) *Vitamins and Hormones*, Vols. 25—27, Academic Press, New York and London (1967—69).
12. Long, C. (Ed.), *Biochemists' Handbook*, Van Nostrand Reinhold, New York (1961).
13. Needham, A. E., *The Growth Process in Animals*, Van Nostrand Reinhold, New York (1964).

14. Oser, B. L. (Ed.), *Hawk's Physiological Chemistry*, 14th Ed., McGraw-Hill (Blakiston Div.), New York (1965).
15. Stecher, P. G. (Ed.), *The Merck Index*, 8th Ed., Merck & Co., Inc., Rahway, N.J. (1968).
16. Weast, R. C. (Ed.), *Handbook of Chemistry and Physics*, 49th Ed., The Chemical Rubber Co., Cleveland, Ohio (1968).
17. West, E. S., Todd, W. R., Mason, H. S., and Van Bruggen, J. T., *Textbook of Biochemistry*, 4th Ed., Macmillan, New York (1966).
18. Williams, R. J. and Lansford, E. M., Jr. (Eds.), *The Encyclopedia of Biochemistry*, Van Nostrand Reinhold, New York (1967).
19. *National Formulary*, XIII Ed., Prepared by National Formulary Board, Am. Pharmaceutical Assoc., Washington, D.C. (1970).
20. *The Pharmacopeia of the United States of America*, 18th Revision, Prepared by the Committee of Revision, The United States Pharmacopeial Convention, Inc., Bethesda, Md. (1971).

Specific: Vitamins

21. Bonner, J. and Varner, J. E. (Eds.), *Plant Biochemistry*, Academic Press, New York and London (1965).
22. Burton, B. T., *The Heinz Handbook of Nutrition*, 2nd Ed., H. J. Heinz Co. (McGraw-Hill), New York (1965).
23. Davidson, S. and Passmore, R., *Human Nutrition and Dietetics*, 4th Ed., Williams & Wilkins, Baltimore, Md. (1969).
24. DeLuca, H. F. and Suttie, J. W. (Eds.), *The Fat-Soluble Vitamins*, Univ. of Wisconsin Press, Madison, Wis. (1970).
25. Furia, T. E. (Ed.), *Handbook of Food Additives*, The Chemical Rubber Co., Cleveland, Ohio (1968).
26. Goodhart, R. S. and Wohl, M. G., *Manual of Clinical Nutrition*, Lea & Febiger, Philadelphia (1964).
27. Goodwin, T. W., *The Biosynthesis of Vitamins and Related Compounds*, Academic Press, London and New York (1963).
28. McCormick, D. B. and Wright, L. D. (Eds.), *Methods in Enzymology*, Vol. XVIII, *Vitamins and Coenzymes*, Parts A–C, Academic Press, New York and London (1970).
29. Morton, R. A. (Ed.), *Fat-Soluble Vitamins*, Pergamon Press, New York (1970).
30. Robinson, F. A., *The Vitamin Co-factors of Enzyme Systems*, Pergamon Press, New York (1966).
31. Rodale, J. I. and Staff, *The Complete Book of Vitamins*, Rodale Books, Inc., Emmaus, Pa. (1971).
32. Sebrell, W. H., Jr., and Harris, R. S. (Eds. Vols. I–V), Gyorgy, P. and Pearson, W. N. (Eds. Vols. VI–VII), *The Vitamins*, 2nd Ed., Vols. I–VII, Academic Press, New York and London (1967).
33. Strohecker, R. and Henning, H. M., *Vitamin Assay Tested Methods*, The Chemical Rubber Co., Cleveland, Ohio (1966).
34. Wagner, A. F. and Folkers, K., *Vitamins and Coenzymes*, Wiley (Interscience Div.), New York (1964).
35. Wohl, M. G. and Goodhart, R. S. (Eds.), *Modern Nutrition in Health and Disease*, 4th Ed., Lea & Febiger, Philadelphia (1968).
36. National Research Council Pub. # 1694, *Recommended Dietary Allowances*, 7th Revised Ed., Printing and Publishing Office, National Academy of Sciences, Washington, D.C. (1968).

Specific: Hormones

37. Back, N., Martini, L. and Paoletti, R. (Eds.), "Pharmacology of Hormonal Polypeptides and Proteins" in *Advances in Exp. Med. Biol.,* Vol. 2, Plenum Press, New York (1968).
38. Briggs, M. H. (Ed.), *Advances in Steroid Biochemistry and Pharmacology*, Vols. 1 and 2, Academic Press, New York and London (1970).
39. Briggs, M. H. and Brotherton, J., *Steroid Biochemistry and Pharmacology*, Academic Press, London and New York (1970).
40. Butt, W. R., *Hormone Chemistry*, Van Nostrand Reinhold, New York (1967).
41. Eisenstein, A. B. (Ed.), *The Adrenal Cortex*, Little, Brown and Co., Boston (1967).
42. Fieser, L. F. and Fieser, M., *Steroids*, Van Nostrand Reinhold, New York (1959).
43. Frieden, E. and Lipner, H., *Biochemical Endocrinology of the Vertebrates*, Prentice-Hall, Englewood Cliffs, N.J. (1971).
44. Gray, C. H. and Bacharach, A. L. (Eds.), *Hormones in Blood*, 2nd Ed., Vols. 1 and 2, Academic Press, London and New York (1967).
45. Heftmann, E. and Mosettig, E., *Biochemistry of Steroids*, Van Nostrand Reinhold, New York (1960).
46. Krüskemper, H. L., *Anabolic Steroids*, Academic Press, New York and London (1968).
47. Litwack, G. (Ed.), *Biochemical Actions*, Vols. I and II, Academic Press, New York and London (1970).
48. Martini, L. and Ganong, W. F. (Eds.), *Neuroendocrinology*, Vols. I and II, Academic Press, New York and London (1967).
49. McKerns, K. W., *Steroid Hormones and Metabolism*, Appleton-Century-Crofts (Meredith Corp.), New York (1969).
50. Sawin, C. T., *The Hormones*, Little, Brown and Co., Boston (1969).
51. Stear, E. B., and Kadish, A. H. (Eds.), *Hormonal Control Systems*, Elsevier, New York (1969).
52. Tepperman, J., *Metabolic and Endocrine Physiology*, 2nd Ed., Year Book Medical Publishers, Chicago (1968).
53. Turner, C. D. and Bagnara, J. T., *General Endocrinology*, 5th Ed., Saunders, Philadelphia (1971).
54. Von Euler, U. S. and Heller, H. (Eds.), *Comparative Endocrinology*, Vols. I and II, Academic Press, New York and London (1963).
55. Williams, R. H. (Ed.), *Textbook of Endocrinology*, 4th Ed., Saunders, Phildelphia (1968).
56. Zarrow, M. X., Yochim, J. M. and McCarthy, J. L., *Experimental Endocrinology*, Academic Press, New York and London (1964).

ITEMIZED TABLE OF REFERENCES[a]

	Vitamins	Hormones
GENERAL INFORMATION		
1. Synonyms	7, 15, 17, 34	1, 7, 15
2. History	15, 17, 18, 34	9, 15, 18, 42, 52
3. Physiological Forms	17, 25 32	9, 44, 55
4. Active Analogs	14, 17, 25, 32	40, 42, 55
5. Inactive Analogs	14, 17, 32	38, 39, 40, 42, 55
6. Antagonists	1, 7, 14, 17, 32	9, 17, 40
7. Synergists	1, 7, 14, 17, 32	9, 17, 40
8. Physiological Functions	4, 14, 22, 32	3, 4, 8, 17, 41, 55
9. Deficiency Diseases	4, 14, 17, 32	3, 14, 17, 55
10. Essentiality	1, 4, 14, 32	1, 9, 53
CHEMISTRY		
1. Structure	1, 8, 16, 17, 24, 29, 30, 32, 34	1, 8, 9, 15, 16, 45
2. Reactions	4, 15, 17, 20, 24, 29, 30, 32, 34	1, 8, 9, 15, 20
3. Properties	1, 7, 15, 16, 19, 24, 29, 30, 32	1, 7, 8, 9, 15, 16, 19, 20, 37
4. Commercial Production	15, 24, 29, 30, 32, 34	9, 15, 40, 42
5. Isolation	9, 24, 29, 30, 32, 34,	40, 42
6. Determination	14, 17, 33	1, 14, 40, 44, 53, 56
DISTRIBUTION AND SOURCES		
1. Occurrence	17, 22, 24, 27, 29, 30, 32, 34	
2. Dietary Sources	4, 8, 12, 22, 24, 27, 29, 30, 32	
MEDICAL AND BIOLOGICAL ROLE		
1. Species	—	1, 53, 54
2. Units	8, 17, 32	8, 9, 14
3. Blood Levels	2, 8, 14, 32	2, 8, 14
4. Requirements	4, 8, 23, 26, 31, 36	—
5. Administration	8, 9, 30, 34	8, 9, 38, 55
6. Factors Affecting Availability or Release	4, 8, 22, 31	1, 3, 4, 50
7. Deficiency	4, 17, 23, 26, 31, 35	1, 3, 4, 53, 55
8. Overdose	4, 17, 24, 29, 30, 32	1, 3, 4, 38, 53, 55
METABOLIC ROLE		
1. Biosynthesis and Production Sites	4, 21, 27, 28	38, 39, 40, 41, 55
2. Storage Areas	8, 9, 17, 32	8, 9, 17

[a] Numbers under Vitamin and Hormone columns refer to those in list of principal references.

ITEMIZED TABLE OF REFERENCES (*cont.*)

	Vitamins	*Hormones*
METABOLIC ROLE (*cont.*)		
3. Blood Carriers	2, 8, 14, 29, 30	2, 8, 40, 44
4. Half-life	8, 9, 29, 30, 32	8, 9, 44
5. Target Tissues	14, 17, 29, 30, 32	1, 3, 38, 40
6. Reactions	5, 14, 17, 28	4, 5, 40, 43, 46, 49, 50, 53
7. Mode of Action	4, 5, 6, 9, 14, 22, 24	3, 4, 5, 8, 9, 17, 47, 51, 55
8. Catabolism	1, 8, 9, 10, 17, 28	1, 9, 40, 43, 49, 50
MISCELLANEOUS		
1. (Other) Vitamins	8, 11, 13, 30	8, 11, 13, 53
2. (Other) Hormones	8, 11, 13, 53	8, 11, 13, 48, 53
3. Unusual Properties	11, 13, 14, 17	46, 48, 53
4. Relationships	11, 13, 38	11, 13, 38

Index

(Entries followed by T denote Tables)